Hydrotherapy in Practice

Hydrotherapy in Practice

Bridget C. Davis Grad Dip Phys HT MCSP

District Physiotherapist, Camberwell Health District, King's College Hospital, London

Ronald A. Harrison Grad Dip Phys HT MCSP

Superintendent Physiotherapist, The Royal National Hospital for Rheumatic Diseases, Bath

Churchill Livingstone

EDINBURGH LONDON MELBOURNE AND NEW YORK 1988

CHURCHILL LIVINGSTONE
Medical Division of Longman Group UK Limited

Distributed in the United States of America by
Churchill Livingstone Inc., 1560 Broadway, New
York, N.Y. 10036, and by associated companies,
branches and representatives throughout the
world.

First published 1988

ISBN 0-443-03062-6

British Library Cataloguing in Publication Data
Davis, Bridget C.
   Hydrotherapy in practice
   1. Hydrotherapy
   I. Title   II. Harrison, Ronald A.
   615.8'53   RM811

Library of Congress Cataloging in Publication Data
Davis, Bridget C.
   Hydrotherapy in practice
   Includes index.
   1. Hydrotherapy.   2. Hospitals—Hydrotherapy
services—Administration.   3. Hospitals—Hydrotherapy
services—Design and construction.   I. Harrison,
Ronald A., 1938—   . II. Title. [DNLM: 1. Facility
Design and Construction. 2. Hydrotherapy. WB 520 D261h]
RM811.D38 1988   615.8'53   87-11720

Produced by Longman Singapore Publishers (Pte) Ltd
Printed in Singapore

Preface

This book is intended for student physiotherapists, for qualified physiotherapists working in hydrotherapy pools and for those involved in the design, equipping and management of such departments.

The chapter on pool design brings together not only the ideas of the authors but also those of many other physiotherapists who were consulted. It is hoped that this will provide help and stimulation to those physiotherapists who find themselves involved in the designing of new hydrotherapy departments.

The chapter 'Spas and spa treatment' was included because many physiotherapists who were consulted, as well as the authors themselves, felt that physiotherapists should know the rationale behind the various modalities which can be used in hydrotherapy establishments and understand the way in which these treatments are given.

In writing this book we have had considerable support and help from a great number of people.

We should like to thank all those superintendent and senior physiotherapists who completed the questionnaires, the results of which provided material used in the preparation of Chapter 1. We should also like to thank physiotherapists who gave their time to discuss the hydrotherapy departments in their hospitals, particularly Frimley Park and Lewisham Hospitals.

Photographs to illustrate techniques are an integral and indispensible part of a physiotherapy text and we are indebted to patients, physiotherapists and students who agreed to be photographed for many of the illustrations in this book.

We are particularly grateful to Dr M. Dewar of the Bioengineering Centre, University College London for his ideas and help at the draft stage of Chapter 7 and for his permission to use material supplied in personal communication.

B. D. wishes to acknowledge and thank Dr Wilhelm Zinn of Bad Ragaz, Switzerland for the unique opportunities and support given in the early development of the techniques in Bad Ragaz.

The authors would also like to thank the following companies for providing photographs and giving permission for their inclusion in this book: Airlines of Glastonbury for Figure 2.3, Arjo Hospital Equipment Ltd of Reading for Figures 1.5, 1.6 and 9.2, Mecanaids Ltd of Gloucester for Figure 1.9, and The Tintometer Ltd of Salisbury for Figures 2.4, 2.5, and 2.6.

We should like to thank the District General Manager, Camberwell Health Authority for permission to use material from the Camberwell Physiotherapy Policy 'Guidelines on the Treatment of AIDS Patients'.

To Gillian Stocks who typed the manuscript and to Martin Beresford-Veale of the Department of Medical Photography, Royal National Hospital for Rheumatic Diseases for all the line drawings and for the photographs excluding those provided by the commercial companies, we record our sincere thanks.

Finally, we thank Mary Emmerson Law and Dinah Bagshaw at Churchill Livingstone for their long-standing patience and for their encouragement and support throughout the prolonged gestation period of this book.

London and Bath, 1988

B. C. D.
R. A. H.

Contents

1. The pool and the department   1

2. Equipping and managing the pool   25

3. Health and safety in the hydrotherapy department   45

4. Basic physical principles applied to pool exercises   53

5. Physiological effects and contra-indications to pool therapy   65

6. Techniques of exercise in water   75

7. Partial weight-bearing and gait re-education   121

8. Treatment of specific conditions   137

9. Spas and spa treatments   171

Index   181

1

The pool and the department

Many physiotherapists will find themselves required to liaise with architects and others in the designing and planning of hydrotherapy departments and for many, this will be a new experience. Unless pool consultants are used, the architect may also be designing his first hydrotherapy pool. The decisions which are taken on design, size and layout will influence the working of the department and treatments for years to come since alterations to a pool will probably be difficult and expensive to make.

It has to be appreciated from the outset that there cannot be a standard design for a hydrotherapy pool and that each individual department should be planned to cater for the number and the types of patient who will need to be treated.

It is with the accurate gathering of this information and the professional interpretation of the data that the physiotherapist provides the architect with the basic facts, and this should be done before any preliminary designs are put forward.

The physiotherapist will probably wish to visit other departments to see their pools and to discuss with the physiotherapists who work in them their particular advantages and disadvantages. Such visits are particularly useful if they can be arranged in company with the architect.

This chapter represents the views of the authors which have been supplemented by the ideas of others who work in established pools, and in addition, it contains information from a survey of thirty hospital pools with regard to size and use.

Staffing should be planned at the same time as the pool is designed and this will be based on the information which has already been assembled on the prospective workload. It is not too early at this stage to plan staffing levels for they may have implications for other managers who will need to plan ahead for possible extra portering or clerical time, and the information should be made available to the relevant heads of departments as soon as it is available. Neglect of this aspect means that there are unfortunately some hydrotherapy pools which cannot be used fully because there are insufficient staff to work them.

POOL PLANT

Most hospital treatment pools will have a water circulating system and, from this point of view, they are smaller versions of public swimming baths. Close to the pool there will be a room in which is housed the basic equipment which is necessary to maintain the pool water in a fit condition for bathing; this equipment is known as the pool plant. A typical plant will consist of a pump, a filter, a heater or heaters and a device for introducing a disinfecting solution into the circulating water.

Figure 1.1 is a simplified diagrammatic representation of an existing hospital pool plant showing the relationship of the various components.

Water leaves the pool at the outlets at A, drawn by the action of one of the pumps at D. The water passes next through the filter E before entering the calorifiers at G. It then flows back into the pool at inlets H after having received a dose of chlorinating agent from the chlorine dosing pump at L.

Maintenance will not, of course, be the concern of the physiotherapist, but a knowledge of the pool plant layout and an under-

Fig. 1.1 Layout of a typical pool 'plant'. A. Pool outlets; B. & C. Air venting tank and pipe; D. Electric circulating pumps; E. Sand/gravel filter; R. Filter—drain valve, for use in 'back-washing'; G. Calorifiers; H. Pool inlets; J. Pool drain; K. Mains connection; L. Chlorinating pump; M. Overflow; N. Drain; T. Thermostats

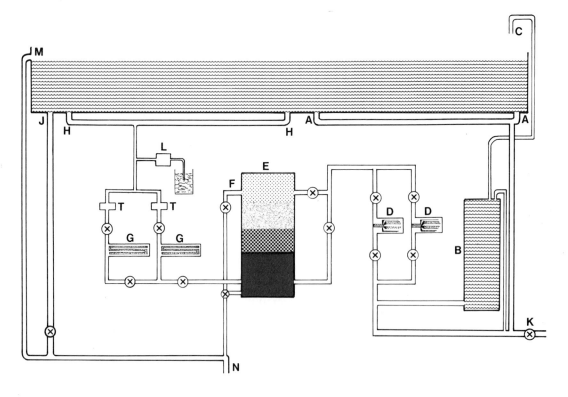

standing of its working is essential, since the engineer's maintenance and repair programme will affect the day-to-day functioning of the pool. The physiotherapist must, therefore, be in a position to discuss with the Works Department, from a position of knowledge, the various options which may be open when maintenance or repairs are necessary. This close co-operation with the engineer is essential if the pool is to be kept in a suitable condition for bathing, and the responsibility for this falls ultimately on the physiotherapist in charge of the hydrotherapy department. When taking charge of a pool the physiotherapist should ask the engineer to show her over the pool plant and ask if, from his point of view, there are any particular difficulties in maintaining it.

Circulating pumps

These will be electrical pumps similar to those on domestic central heating, with which most people are familiar but they are, of course, larger and more powerful. Although only one pump is used at a time, there are usually two provided which are connected into the system in parallel. Valves are positioned so that either pump may be isolated from the circulating system which enables servicing and repairs to be carried out without interrupting the circulation of the treatment pool water.

The size of the pumps, and thus their capacity, determines the rate at which the water circulates. The time taken for a volume of water equivalent to the capacity of the pool to pass through the filter is known as the 'turn-over' time. If the pool is to remain clear and clean it is usually recommended that this time does not exceed four hours and ideally should be less.

Dosing pumps

Agents used for disinfecting the water in the treatment pool are usually introduced in liquid form by means of a small electrically driven pump which injects measured doses of the solution into circulating water continuously over the twenty-four hours. This arrangement keeps the level of the disinfecting agent constant, replacing it as it is used. Each dose consists of only a few millilitres, but since the pump works continuously at a rate of about eight hundred strokes per hour, over a period of twenty-four hours many gallons of the solution will be introduced into the pool. The solution is stored in a tank which will contain about twenty or thirty gallons and is replenished regularly by the engineer.

Both the rate of pumping and volume injected at each stroke can be easily adjusted by the engineer if this is indicated by a consistently inappropriate level of disinfecting agent. Once a setting for a particular pool which has a regular bathing load has been established, further adjustment of the pump will probably be indicated very rarely.

These pumps are reliable in use and seem to give little trouble if properly serviced. Where sodium hypochlorite solution is used regular cleaning of the pump and the narrow injection pipe are necessary since the hypochlorite crystallises out and can block the pipe, and this results in a rapid drop in the chlorine level in the pool. The routine cleaning of the injection pipe can usually be done by the engineer without any interruption of the functioning of the treatment pool.

Calorifiers

The function of the calorifiers or heaters is to add a small quantity of heat to the water as it circulates, to compensate for the heat which is lost from the pool surface and from the pipework, etc. For this reason they are not usually large enough to heat large quantities of water quickly. This may give the physiotherapist organisational problems after emptying and refilling the pool and again this emphasises the necessity for close co-operation with the 'works staff' on deciding the timing of maintenance and repair jobs. Just as the circulating pumps are often provided as a pair, in parallel, this is often the case with calorifiers, only one of the pair being in use most of the time. This enables servicing, repairs and periodic insurance checks of the calorifiers to be carried out without interruption of the normal working of the pool.

Both calorifiers may be used when it is necessary to bring the temperature of the pool up quickly, e.g. after re-filling or 'back washing' the filter.

Calorifiers usually consist of a large copper cylinder through which the circulating pool water passes. As it does so it flows over a system of pipes through which steam or hot water is flowing from the hospital boilers and the pool water is thus heated by a simple heat exchange. The calorifiers are fitted with thermostats which once set should keep the temperature of the pool water within acceptable limits.

Filters

Dust and debris are continously introduced into every pool no matter what precautions are taken. Every time a bather enters the water, small amounts of epidermis, hair and 'lint' from costumes will find their way into the water. In addition to this there is the fine dust in the air which settles on the pool surface. If the treatment pool is to remain clear and clean this foreign matter must be removed from the water continuously and an efficient filter is, therefore, an essential component of the pool plant and the pool water should pass through it reasonably often (see 'turn-over time', p. 3).

There are several types of filter in use in hospital pools and the physiotherapist should be aware of the type in use in her pool.

The types of filter are:
1. Sand and gravel filter
2. Diatomaceous earth filter
3. Disposable cartridge filter.

Sand and gravel filter

This type of filter is commonly used for hospital pools and it consists of a large metal cylinder into which are packed layers of sand and gravel which trap the foreign particles as the water passes through the various layers. These layers of sand and gravel are known as the filter 'bed' and may consist of up to six graded layers ranging from pieces of gravel 2 cm in diameter to a layer of fine sharp sand. Some pools may have a 'strainer box' through which the water passes before it goes to the filter and this will remove the larger pieces of debris.

Diatomaceous earth filter

This is essentially a rechargeable filter and whereas in the gravel filter the 'bed' is washed, in this type of filter it is replaced after each backwash, the 'bed' being washed away to waste with the dirt. The bed of this type is a powdery substance, but is in fact, composed of a naturally occurring material composed of the silicaceous remains of marine organisms called diatoms. The powder is supported in the filter on a very fine mesh of man-made fibre.

Disposable cartridge filter

This is an expensive method of filtering when used in a hospital pool. The filter consists of an element which is thrown away when it is no longer working efficiently. These cartridges are made of pads of bonded fibre and foam and cannot be cleaned. The authors know of only one hospital pool where this method is used.

'Back-washing'

Obviously if a filter performs its function efficiently and removes the solid debris from the circulating pool water, then a time will be reached when the filter will become effectively blocked by the dirt trapped in the filter 'bed' and the filter will no longer function. This must not be allowed to happen and, therefore, one of the regular maintenance tasks of the engineer will be to clean the filter by the process generally known as 'back-washing'. This is simply a reversal of the flow of water through the filter 'bed' which lifts out the dirt as well as loosening the bed so that it does not become solid. The dirty water containing the debris lifted from the bed is allowed to run to waste in the main drain.

Back-washing will be carried out at frequent intervals on a regular basis, but the frequency will vary according to the needs of a particular pool. It may in some circumstances be necessary to back-wash the filter daily or it may only be required once per week. This will depend upon the type and size of the filter. A relatively small filter will require attention more frequently than a larger filter, given the same sized pools, since it will become blocked more quickly.

The water used for the back-washing is usually taken from the pool and, therefore, the level in the pool will drop whilst this is taking place. After back-washing the pool level will be made up by the addition of clean water and, therefore, at every back-wash a proportion of the pool water is changed. Since it is unlikely that the water used to top up the pool will be at the same temperature as the circulating water some variation in temperature may be expected. If the filter is large and a large volume of water is needed for the back-wash which is then made up by using cold mains water, the physiotherapist will need to arrange a mutually convenient time if treatment is not to be interrupted whilst the pool is reheated.

DISINFECTION OF TREATMENT POOL WATER

Since the water in the treatment pool may not be completely changed for periods varying from several weeks to a year, it must be continously disinfected if it is to remain free of pathogenic and other organisms. Traditionally the water in public swimming pools and in hospital pools has been treated by the use of chlorine, although the method of introduction of chlorine to the water has varied. Although chlorine is probably still the most commonly used agent, the physiotherapist must be prepared to find other disinfecting agents in use in hydrotherapy pools.

Chlorine

Until recently the method of choice for public swimming bath chlorination was the use of gaseous chlorine. Chlorine in a cylinder was fed through a chlorinator which dissolved measured amounts of chlorine in water and injected it into the circulating pool water. This method was occasionally used in the larger hospital pools, but it is more usual to find that the chlorine is introduced as a soluble compound which releases the chlorine when it is in solution. Such compounds are known as 'chlorine donors'. Examples of chlorine donors are:
1. Sodium hypochlorite
2. Calcium hypochlorite
3. Chloro-iso-cyanurate.

Sodium hypochlorite

This is household or laundry bleach and is usually obtained under the trade names of Chloros or Bridos. It is probably still the commonest agent used for the chlorination of hospital treatment pools. When purchased it has a chlorine content of approximately 15% w/w of available chlorine, but is diluted before it is fed into the pool mechanically by means of a pump (see 'dosing pump', p. 3).

Occasionally in older hospital pools there may be no facility for introducing the sodium hypochlorite mechanically, and one may be reduced to treating the pool by pouring the disinfecting agent directly into the pool. This is known as 'hand chlorination' and is a rather hit and miss method which carries problems which will be discussed later (p. 43).

Calcium hypochlorite

This is a dry form of chlorine donor being available in crystalline or in tablet form. It is said to have 65% available chlorine w/w and to be 95% soluble.

Chloro-iso-cyanurates

These substances were originally developed commercially as compounds for use in laundry products, but are now used for the chlorination of pools. This agent can be obtained as granules for 'hand-chlorination', the granules dissolving completely as they fall through the water leaving no sediment and giving off available chlorine.

Iso-cyanurates can also be obtained as tablets which are hung in a plastic container in the pool and dissolve slowly over a day or two giving a steady release of available chlorine. Iso-cyanurates may also be introduced automatically via a dosing pump after they have been dissolved in water.

Bromine

Bromine occurs in the Periodic Table of elements in the same position as chlorine, both of them belonging to the group of elements called halogens. As would be expected, therefore, they have similar chemical properties and bromine is sometimes used as a disinfecting agent in swimming and treatment pools. Just as gaseous chlorine can be dangerous, bromine in its elemental form is a hazardous substance to handle and safer compounds have been developed for the treatment of water. Di-halo is a solid form of bromine in combination with some chlorine and is obtained in the form of rods which are placed in a sealed glass unit through which a controlled flow of water passes, carrying with it the dissolved bromine. This method of disinfecting treatment pool water is used in some hospital pools, but it may be worth noting that there is strong circumstantial evidence for the association of this type of pool treatment with dermatoses which are mainly of an eczematous nature (Rycroft and Penny 1983).

Baquacil

A few hospital pools are now using this material to treat their water. It represents a complete break with the traditional use of halogens. Baquacil is not an oxidising agent and does have some attractions to the small pool user. Baquacil is added to the pool until a concentration of fifty parts per million is reached and then no further addition is necessary until the level falls to twenty-five parts per million. Every four weeks, however, hydrogen peroxide must be added. If this agent is used the maker's instructions must be followed exactly as its efficacy may be affected by the addition of other substances, e.g. chlorine, some algicides.

Ozone

Ozone is a powerful disinfectant, but compared with other methods tends to be expensive. It has the disadvantage that ozone residuals tend to disappear quickly, thus making it difficult to maintain a threshold. For this reason, where it has been used in Britain, supplementary halogen treatment has been used (Humphrey 1978).

VENTILATION

It is by means of an adequate ventilating system that the comfortable working environment of the physiotherapist and patients is maintained. Two of the main factors which contribute to the thermal comfort of an individual are the air temperature and the humidity, and since the pool acts, in effect, as a large radiator and humidifier it presents rather special problems from the point of view of environment. Problems may arise from time to time and it is important that the physiotherapist should have some understanding of the principles of ventilation.

Extracting ventilating system

This is a simple system whereby air is withdrawn from the room by mechanical means, i.e. extractor fans. The air which replaces that which has been extracted, finds its own way into the room via cracks, doorways, windows or through specially prepared apertures called 'fresh air inlets'. If this type of ventilation is used, the physiotherapist must be aware of the possibility that there may be some places in the department where there are draughts, and procedures should be organised so that unclothed patients are not required to be in these areas.

Plenum ventilating system

This is a system where air is blown into the room from outside and the air which is displaced finds its way out through the doors, windows, etc. The disadvantage of this system in a hydrotherapy department is that the warm, humid air might very well be pushed out into other treatment areas where these adjoin the pool room.

Balanced ventilating system

This is really a combination of the first two systems whereby fresh air is blown into the room by one set of fans, whilst air is extracted by another set. This arrangement gives a fair measure of control of ventilation and is used successfully in many hospital hydrotherapy departments.

Air conditioning

Air conditioning is a system of ventilation which adjusts automatically the temperature and the humidity of the environment. A central 'plant' keeps the quality of the air within predetermined limits by cooling or heating, humidifying or dehumidifying and cleaning it, as well as moving it around the building.

Fresh air is drawn into the building from outside and mixed with a proportion of the air which has already been circulated. The addition of recirculated air reduces heat loss and thus relieves the load on the conditioning plant. It will be appreciated that with extractor and balanced ventilation the air which is extracted to waste carries with it heat. With the increasing cost of fuel for heating, recirculation of air which is already warm has economic advantages.

Some two hundred large municipal swimming pools have, over the last few years, installed heat reclamation systems, but unfortunately there now seems to be strong evidence that this type of system is associated with attacks of bronchospasm. This is said to be due to the fact that air recirculation concentrates some of the chlorine compounds in the air, and nitrogen trichloride has been suggested as the chemical responsible. The asthmatic bather is particularly susceptible, but bronchial wheezing has been noted in non-asthmatics (Penny 1983).

It has to be said that as yet there are few small hospital pools with air conditioning, but the physiotherapist should be aware of this possible effect of air conditioning where heat reclamation systems are installed.

POOL SIZE

In the hydrotherapy departments' survey, the sizes of pools varied a great deal, and this variation is illustrated in Figure 1.2, where the sizes are represented by surface area. From this it can be seen that approximately 30% of the pools had areas which were between 15 m² and 20 m². This figure compares closely with the 32% which Greenless found for this size of pool in a survey of British hydrotherapy pools (Skinner and Thomson 1983).

The five pools which users complained were too small are represented on the histogram by the dotted blocks and are all pools below the surface area of 15 m². The physiotherapists in charge of these pools indicated that not only was the number of treatments limited, but also that the quality of their treatments was decreased because they were not able to use some techniques because of the inadequate dimensions of the pool.

Unfortunately, from the physiotherapist's point of view, it has been shown that pool area is the most important factor determining the cost of a pool room (The Sports Council).

Several departments in the survey had originally been intended, in the early planning stages, to have larger pools than were eventually built. This was because of financial restraints which became apparent as the planning proceeded, and money was saved by decreasing the dimensions of the pool.

It may be useful for the physiotherapist to know, if such circumstances arise, that the third most important factor determining the cost is the depth of the water. Serious thought should be given to deciding what is the minimum depth that will be satisfactory in that particular case. It may be that a small saving on depth may enable the physiotherapist to have a marginally larger pool.

Fig. 1.2 Results of a survey of pool size of thirty hospital hydrotherapy pools

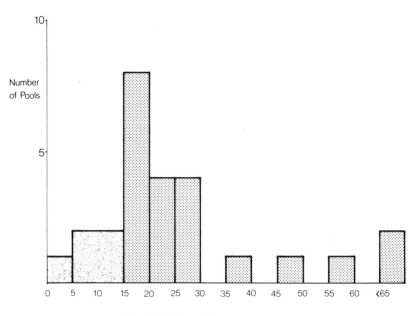

Pool area in Square Metres

On the other hand, it may be possible that some refinement in the fitting of the pool room may be sacrificed to maintain pool size in the hope that money may be available at a later date to make good the deficit.

Certainly pools having areas which are considered by the physiotherapists working in them to be too deep for treatment are not hard to find, and the money wasted on providing an inappropriate depth of water could have been used to increase the usable area of the pool.

The authors favour a rectangular pool with a minimum length of 6 m and a minimum width of 4 m.

POOL DEPTH

The optimum depth of a hydrotherapy pool for the majority of treatments which are carried out on adult patients will be equal to the waist or mid-chest height of the physiotherapist. Such a depth will make for ease of handling the patient in the floating position and at the same time will not give rise to difficulties in maintaining balance and 'foothold' whilst resisting the patients' movements, stabilising or providing fixation.

In practice, a depth of between 1.0 m and 1.2 m will be suitable for most physiotherapists. It is usually considered that some areas of the pool should be provided with depths less than and greater than this optimum, for use with children or for the progression of walking re-education, etc.

If, after considering the type of patient to be treated, it is felt that a pool with varying depth is needed, one must consider which of the various methods of achieving this is most suitable for the particular situation.

The options open to the pool designer are:
1. Sloping floor
2. Stepped floor
3. Combination of steps and sloping floor

Sloping floor

This is the traditional way in which varying depth has been provided in swimming pools and the idea was naturally transferred to treatment pools when these began to be built in hospitals. Generally, however, hydrotherapy pools are much smaller than swimming pools and accommodating the variation in depth required in small pools results in slopes which are not suitable for some aspects of treatment. The most obvious of these is walking re-education, for even a slope of 1:20 will have the effect on a patient equal to that of 1.5 cm leg shortening when he is walking across the slope of the pool. Where walking re-education is a substantial part of the treatment to be carried out, it would seem desirable to provide at least some areas with a level bottom.

Stepped pools

This type of pool has two or more level lanes of differing depths which are separated from each other by steps. The lanes usually run the length of the pool. This arrangement offers a solution to the problem stated above and is one which has been adopted by many designers of hydrotherapy pools.

It is sometimes suggested that stepped pools could be dangerous and that rails should be fitted between the lanes to prevent patients stepping inadvertently into deeper water. The experience of most physiotherapists who have worked in this type of pool does not support this idea. If the edges of the lanes are picked out in different coloured tiles and if the patients are adequately instructed and supervised, there is no necessity to fit rails and the steps do not constitute a danger.

Figure 1.3 shows a cross-section of an existing pool of this type. In this particular pool, children are not treated, and although the shallow lane is not really deep enough for treatment in the standing position it has been utilised by the provision of a weighted stool so that patients may sit in this lane whilst performing shoulder exercises. The steps for patients entering the pool over the wall are also in this lane.

Fig. 1.3 Shallow lane of a stepped pool. A, Weighted stool. B, Steps

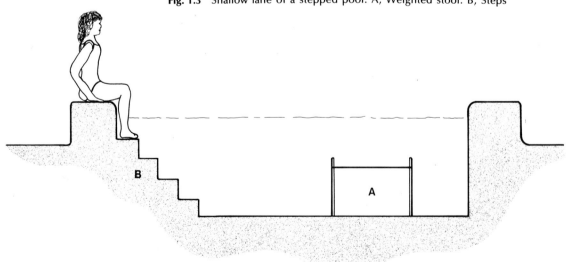

Combination of steps and slope

The authors know of only one hydrotherapy pool which has this design: the pool having two level lanes of different depths sandwiched between three bands of sloping floor. This hydrotherapy pool is large by hospital standards and it is because of this that such an arrangement is possible. Physiotherapists who work in this pool find this to be an entirely satisfactory solution.

Built in seat/shelf

One pool in the survey had a built-in shelf which was of a suitable height for adult patients to sit whilst doing shoulder exercises, but was also used as a shallow walking lane for small children. This is an idea which others may find useful where provision for children has to be made and pool size is limited.

BAYS AND GLASS SIDED POOLS

It is the opinion of the authors that treatment by hydrotherapy can only be carried out satisfactorily when the physiotherapist is in the water with the patient. Some treatments can be carried out from the side of the pool, but they must of necessity be limited by the fact that many useful techniques will not be possible.

Two variations of pool design have been used as an aid to directing exercises from outside the pool:

1. Bays

The construction of a bay or 'dry dock' is essentially the provision of a dry area in which the physiotherapist may stand at the same level as the level of the patient. As has been pointed out this arrangement allows treatment from outside the pool, but without the need for steps over a raised wall (Bolton and Goodwin 1983).

Figure 1.4 illustrates such a bay which was formerly used at the Hot Springs Physical Treatment Centre, Bath.

Fig. 1.4 'Dry dock' or treatment bay

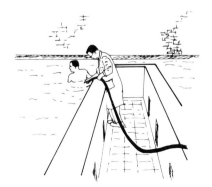

2. Glass-sided pools

Such pools enable the physiotherapist on the outside of the pool to observe the movements of the lower limbs during exercise and walking re-education (see Fig. 1.5).

HOISTS

All hydrotherapy departments which treat the physically disabled will need a hoist with which to lift patients in and out of the pool with the minimum of discomfort to the patients and the maximum safety to the helpers.

Hoists may be fitted with stretchers or with chairs and some models are made so that these are interchangeable.

Pool lifts are powered by different means and this gives a convenient way of classifying them:

1. Hydraulic hoists
2. Electrical hoists
3. Mechanical hoists
4. Compressed air hoists.

Hydraulic (Fig. 1.6)

These hoists consist essentially of a large piston which is powered by water pressure from the cold water mains supply. The principle by which these hoists work can be illustrated by referring to Figure 1.7, which represents two pistons which are free to move in their sleeves. The two piston chambers and the pipe connecting them are filled with water. Chamber 1 has a cross-sectional area of 10 cm, whilst chamber 2 has a cross-sectional area of 1 cm.

Fig. 1.5 The 'Arjo' glass-sided pool. (Reproduced with permission from Arjo Hospital Equipment Ltd 1986)

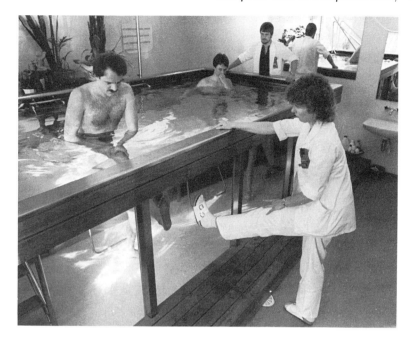

Fig. 1.6 The 'Arjo' hydraulic pool hoist. (Reproduced with permission from Arjo Hospital Equipment Ltd 1986)

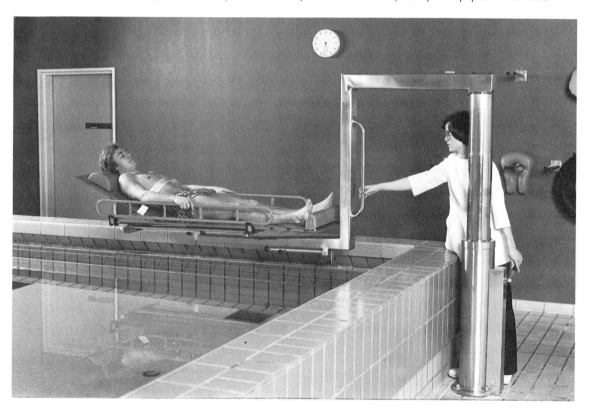

Since the pressure throughout the water is the same, a weight of 10 kg resting on piston 1 will cause a pressure of 1 kg/sq cm on both chambers. A weight of 1 kg is sufficient, therefore, when resting on piston 2 to counterbalance the 10 kg weight. If the 1 kg weight is replaced by a 2 kg weight the piston in chamber 2 will descend and the 10 kg weight will be raised (Fig. 1.7).

It is by using this principle that the pressure in the cold water mains can be used to lift the weight of stretcher and patient.

Operation (Fig. 1.8)

The hoist is usually fitted with two taps; one marked 'raise' and the other 'lower'.

1. When the 'raise' tap is opened, water from the mains flows into chamber A and the pressure forces the piston upwards carrying with it the hoist arm and the stretcher. During this time the 'lower' tap must be closed.

2. When the 'lower' tap is opened and the 'raise' tap is closed, the water from chamber A flows out and is lost down the drain. The weight of the piston, stretcher and patient pushes the water out of chamber A, but because the pipe through which it is forced has such a narrow bore it can escape only slowly and the stretcher descends gently.

NB. At no time should both taps be open at the same time and when the hoist is stationary, either in the raised or lowered position, both taps should be closed.

Faulty seals

The working of the hydraulic hoist depends upon the integrity of the seals and the various moving parts being water-tight. If the seals are faulty air may be sucked into the system or water may leak out and the hoist will not work correctly. The metal piston has one, or sometimes two, leather or plastic inserts which ensure an exact and water-tight fit between the piston and the wall of the chamber.

If these seals become worn then they must be replaced or the hoist will not function efficiently.

A common sign that the seals may be worn is when the lift works in a jerky manner. This is probably a sign that there is air in the piston chamber. The hoist is provided with a valve for bleeding air from the piston chamber in the same way that central heating radiators are 'bled' and this may need to be done from time to time. When the seals are worn this will need to be done more frequently by the hospital engineer who may suggest that a date should be fixed for the hoist to be stripped down and overhauled.

Hydraulic hoists when not in use should be kept at their lowest level.

Fig. 1.7 Diagrammatic representation of the hydraulic principle

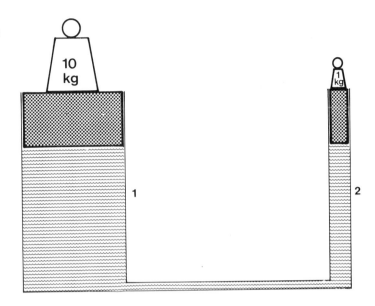

Fig. 1.8 Section through a hydraulic hoist

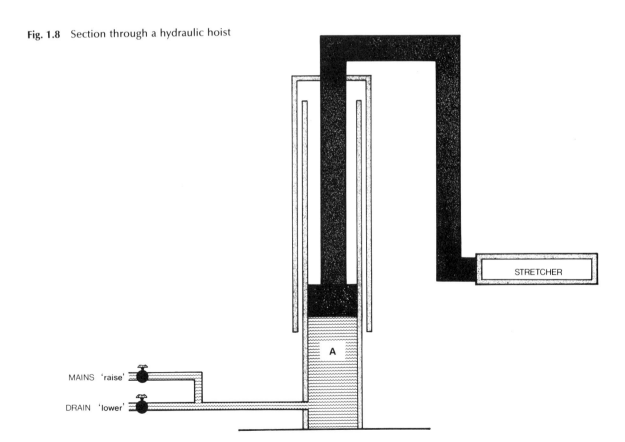

Faulty washers

The 'raise' and 'lower' taps on the hydraulic hoist are similar to domestic taps on a sink and, like sink taps, can develop worn washers. Signs that the washers are leaking are:

1. Slower than normal operation when raising the hoist.
2. The hoist slowly lowering itself from the fully-raised position although both the taps are closed.

Replacing a washer is a few minutes' job for the fitter, but fitting new seals on the piston will take an hour or two and will have to be arranged in advance if treatment sessions are not to be interfered with.

Both of these faults make themselves known slowly and complete failure occurring suddenly would be very unusual. This means that the physiotherapist in charge of the hydrotherapy department should be able to plan ahead with the engineer or fitter for the necessary work to be done without disrupting the patients' treatment times.

Electrical hoists

These are similar in many ways to the electrical hoists which are fitted in disabled patients' homes. The electric motor which powers the lifting mechanism travels on an overhead trackway which is suspended from a specially strengthened ceiling.

The movement of the stretcher from the side of the pool to a position over the water may be electrically powered or the hoist may be moved manually by the operator. The patient is carried either in canvas or nylon slings or on a seat. A stretcher is also available for those patients unable to sit or who are unsafe in that position. Some patients are apprehensive about not only being raised off their wheelchair, but also carried forward on the gantry over the pool before being lowered. It is necessary, therefore, to ensure that pool-side helpers do not raise the patient too high before moving him forwards over the pool.

Mechanical (Fig. 1.9)

A mechanical hoist is similar in design to a hydraulic hoist, having an upright post fixed into the floor, and movable side beam with chair or stretcher. The means of transferring the patient into the water is by winding to raise the chair, then swinging the beam so that the patient is over the pool. The beam is then locked in position, the mechanism is wound in the reverse direction and so the patient is lowered into the water.

As there is no connection to a water supply the upright post can be fitted in such a way that it can be removed from the floor and a cover placed over the hole. This facility is perhaps more useful in a swimming pool where disabled swimmers require a hoist for access to the water. However, in certain pool departments it is also an advantage to be able to remove the hoist.

These hoists are simple in operation and give a smooth ride.

Fig. 1.9 The 'Mecanaids' pool lift. (Reproduced with permission from Mecanaids Ltd Gloucester 1986)

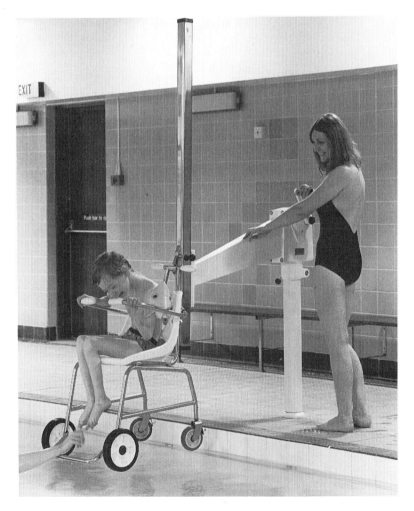

Compressed air hoists

These hoists are met with only occasionally in hydrotherapy departments. They consist of a torpedo-shaped cylinder which travels along a suspended trackway from the poolside out over the water in a similar fashion to an electrical hoist.

Within the cylinder is a piston to which is attached, via a set of pulleys, a strong wire cable. The end of this cable comes out of the base of the cylinder and terminates in a large weighted hook. To this hook is attached a specially designed chair.

To raise the chair a button is pressed which allows compressed air to enter the cylinder and push the piston which in turn draws the cable inside. To lower the chair another button is pressed and the air escapes in a rather noisy manner when compared with the operation of other types of hoist. The operator's pressure on the buttons determines the speed at which the chair moves up and down.

OTHER FACILITIES

Utility room

Adjacent to or opening out of the pool area, will be the utility room. It is here that there are facilities for washing, rinsing, drying and airing bathing costumes as well as for disinfecting footwear. A large deep sink is necessary, also a washing machine, spin-drier and rack or line for airing damp costumes. The size of this area, although dependent upon space available, should be approximately 2.2 m by 3.2 m.

Changing cubicles

Six changing cubicles need to be available for patients and need to be at least 2 m by 1 m. A wide fixed bench must be provided and grab-rails are useful. Depending upon the space available for changing cubicles it may be possible to provide lockers in each cubicle for the patient's clothes. An alternative is to provide wire baskets such as are used in some swimming pools. When undressed, the patient places his clothes and all belongings in the basket and gives it to the helper who places it in a designated secure area.

In addition to these changing cubicles a larger curtained area is necessary so that patients unable to stand can be undressed on a stretcher or bed before entering the pool area.

A suggested layout for such an area in the form of a cubicle has been given by Walter (1971). It contains a WC suite, a wash-hand basin, and a shower facility. Grab-rails are fixed to the wall and there is a rail for the WC. The floor area is approximately 5.11 m.

Toilets

In the hydrotherapy department it is recommended that there are two toilets, one male and one female. A third toilet with wide access suitable for a patient in a wheelchair should be available for the disabled of both sexes. If space is available a toilet should also be provided for staff.

Rest area

Some patients for whom pool therapy is useful become easily fatigued (particularly those with a systemic condition), and these patients should rest immediately after the pool session. A rest room should, therefore, be available with an air temperature of approximately 18.5 °C. A divan bed is provided on which the patient can rest having been packed in a sheet, towel and blankets for twenty to thirty minutes. Half-way through the rest period the pack is loosened and the top blanket removed. The purpose of resting the patient in this manner is to allow the heart rate, blood pressure and body temperature to return to normal whilst the patient is not exerting himself in any way. Following the rest period the patient dresses himself and must be provided with a drink to counteract fluid loss (see p. 66).

Staff base

Within the pool area it will be necessary to have a desk or table where an attendance book can be kept as well as current patients' notes, and where records and reports can be written. Here also the schedule for pool sessions is kept. An appointments board which has been found most useful in pool departments is the type with a plastic surface which can be wiped clean. Fibre tipped pens with water soluble ink are used and, therefore, names are easily written and easily read.

A telephone should also be at the staff base, not least in order that help can be summoned in the event of an emergency.

Alarm system

It is essential that there is some means of summoning help from the pool. This is necessary in cases of emergency so that the physiotherapist in the pool may call other staff to assist the helper. The helper cannot always be at the pool-side for she will be receiving patients, sorting laundry, rinsing and drying costumes, assisting patients in the changing cubicles and performing many other tasks in the hydrotherapy department. The system found to be most efficient is that of a cord hanging over the pool which the therapist can pull and thus sound the alarm. If the pool is large then it is useful to have two or even three pull cords.

Shower and footbath

Shower

There must be a shower in the pool area close to the point of entry to the pool. When undressed and in his bathing costume the patient is escorted to the shower under which he should stand or sit for at least one minute. The purpose of this is two-fold: firstly for hygienic purposes, rinsing off dust particles, and secondly, to prepare the patient for entry into the warm pool. The temperature of the shower should be neutral, around 35 °C, and should be controlled by a thermostatic mixing valve.

Leonard thermostatic mixing valve

The valve has two functions:
1. To keep the water blended and at required temperature.
2. To act as a safety device to prevent scalding of the patient by full hot output in the event of failure of the cold water supply acting as a 'fail-safe' device.

The valve has two controls, thermostatic and manual.

Operation

Water control is turned fully on and the temperature control (or degree of warmth) is turned to the required temperature. As the temperature control is turned, so the port sleeve slides over the port pillar opening the ports to allow hot water into the valve. If the temperature within the mixing chamber becomes too hot, a metallic strip expands and as this is wound in a spiral fashion it turns the spindle and, therefore, also the port sleeve to close down the ports on the hot side and at the same time increases the amount of cold water entering the valve by opening the cold water ports.

Footbath

Ideally the footbath should be sited at the bottom of the steps into the pool and built into the floor. It does not need to be deep (approximately 10 cm) and a suggested size of 50 cm by 50 cm would be suitable. The footbath should contain a 1% solution of chloros, hexachlorathene or other suitable disinfectant. All patients and staff should pass through the footbath before entry into the pool.

HAND RAILS

Hand rails at the pool steps

Although the patient who is unsteady on his feet will be assisted by a helper on the outside of the pool and will be received into the pool by the phyiotherapist, provision of a hand rail at the steps is essential. The minimum diameter of such rails should be 50 mm so that those patients unable to make a fist can still hold them satisfactorily.

Hand rails within the pool

Some pools have been built with no hand rail within the pool, and the only fixation that the patient can take from the wall is gained by holding on to the edge of the 'scum channel'. This is not really satisfactory and it makes impossible the use of many very useful starting positions. A hand rail of at least 50 mm diameter and offset from the wall can be considered to be an item of equipment.

The attention of the architect should be drawn to the fact that it will be used as such so that provision is made in the construction for the rail to take the strains which will from time to time be placed upon it. These may be quite considerable if one imagines, for example, four or five members of a back class all taking fixation from the rail whilst doing strong trunk exercises.

If a scum channel is incorporated in addition to the hand rail, care must be taken in their relative positioning so that it is not possible for a foot to become jammed under the rail with the heel in the channel when this starting position is used (Walter 1971).

FLOORING

The use of correct flooring materials in a pool department is of extreme importance, and costs are high if flooring has to be replaced subsequent to original building. Much has been written about suitable flooring and the architect will be familiar with the latest materials (Walter 1971).

The pool

It may seem unnecessary to remind physiotherapists that the floor of the pool should be of non-slip tiles, but it has to be said that there are some hydrotherapy pools where this has been over-looked. A non-slip surface is necessary not only to prevent accidental slipping, but also because the physiotherapist must have a firm grip on the bottom to resist the patient's efforts and to give counter-resistance to strengthening exercises, etc. Pools with glazed tile floors make the provision of counter-resistance to vigorous exercises impossible.

One of the pools in the survey had non slip-tiles with a deep relief pattern which was uncomfortable to the feet and walking re-education with rheumatoids was not possible. As has been pointed out by Walter (1971) such tiles also present a hazard to those patients with deficient skin sensation or poor skin such as paraplegics and spina bifida patients.

The pool-side area including shower

The floor should have an effective fall towards suitably positioned grids to assist in the cleaning of the floor and also to ensure that any surface water is disposed of rapidly. The floor in this area will be constantly wet due to the passage of patients and staff to and from the pool and the accidental splashing from the pool. It is, therefore, potentially a real hazard. The tiling in this area should be of a non-slip variety, but where they are fitted around a sunken pool the particular pattern should be chosen carefully. It may be that with such a pool the physiotherapist may wish to bring patients into the pool from the sides and this may require the patient to lie on the edge of the pool.

Patients with poor skin such as those with spina bifida or paraplegics could damage themselves if tiles with a too deep relief pattern were used.

The area immediately around the hoist is a particularly 'wet' area and it is often not appreciated how much water drips from the stretcher and the patient onto the floor each time it is used. A drain beneath the stretcher is essential, for it is precisely in this area where patients are being lifted and handled that there should be a safe non-slip surface. Provision of a drain at this point will obviate the necessity for constant 'mopping up' during treatment sessions.

Changing cubicle area

A non-slip floor is also important here, as patients walk into the changing area immediately after having showered and are therefore, still wet. Usually it is possible to have a non-slip vinyl flooring, although many departments continue the non-slip ceramic tiling through to this area.

REFERENCES

Bolton E, Goodwin D 1983 Benefits of new pool design. Therapy November 24
Harris R 1963 Therapeutic pools. In: Lichts (ed) Medical hydrology. Waverley Press, Maryland
Humphrey W H, 1978 Public swimming pool water disinfection. Royal Society of Health Journal 98: 22–24
Skinner A T, Thomson A M 1983 Duffield's exercise in water. Balliere Tindall, London, p 24
The Sports Council 1975 Building cost study of 25 m indoor swimming pools. Technical Unit for Sport Bulletin 3, The Sports Council, London
Walter F 1971 Sports centres and swimming pools. The Thistle Foundation, Edinburgh

2

Equipping and managing the pool

Relatively little equipment is required for a hydrotherapy department apart from a hoist. The larger items consist of submerged plinths, stools and parallel bars, and the smaller equipment includes all flotation aids, balls, paddles, weighted sandals, etc.

LARGE EQUIPMENT

Submerged plinths

A plinth allows for fixation of the patient and many physiotherapists find them to be of great advantage, particularly for the patient who is severely paralysed or who is in a lot of pain. The most common type of plinth is one which can be hooked over the edge of the pool or over the hand rail to lie at an angle just below the surface of the water (Fig. 2.1).

Fig. 2.1 Submerged half-plinth

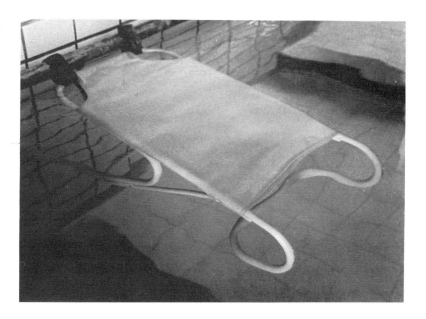

There are usually one or two slings of canvas or nylon which lend support to the upper trunk. The patient can be provided with a support for the head, and if able he can hold the sides of the plinth for fixation. Alternatively, either a strap can be placed around the patient's pelvis or he can be fixed manually by the physiotherapist. Another type of plinth is one in which there are two submerged parallel bars fixed into the floor of the pool. Between the bars are two canvas or nylon slings, a head support is provided and the patient fixed in the way previously described.

There is an advantage in having a movable plinth as it can be taken out of the pool when space is needed for other activities. It is a good rule in fact to have no fixed equipment in the pool if movable equivalent equipment can be obtained.

Submerged stools

These are commonly made of wood, although sometimes of stainless steel. Occasionally, a seating facility will be built as an integral part of the pool. This, however, is not advisable as being permanently in place it reduces the availability of extra space as and when required.

Wooden stools must be made of teak or some other hard wood that does not warp, crack or splinter. The stool should have a slotted seat and will need to be weighted to ensure stability in the water. Depending upon the depth of the water in which it is placed, the stool should be of a height that allows the shoulders of the seated patient to be just below the surface of the water. As a rough guide, if the stool is positioned in water one metre in depth, the seat should be approximately 40 cm off the floor of the pool, but stools are best 'tailor-made' to fit the individual pool. If the hospital works department are willing to make them they can be made of stainless steel.

Parallel bars

It is extremely valuable to have parallel bars in the pool, so that gait activities and other exercises can be given to full advantage. The area of the pool designated for gait activities is usually the deepest part where the water is four feet or more in depth. Provision of parallel bars can be made sometimes by using the hand rail of the pool on one side, and therefore only one extra bar is required. Bars should be of stainless steel or some other material which will not corrode or rust and it is not necessary for parallel bars to be adjustable in height.

Parallel bars which are fixed by uprights into a platform which can be raised and lowered in the water are felt by some physiotherapists to be very useful, particularly if any children are treated in the pool as well as adults.

Hand rail

A hand rail, preferably of stainless steel, should be attached all around the pool at the level of the surface of the water.

A second rail placed lower down is very useful, particularly for exercises in which the patient is in the side lying position and holding onto the rail. By being able to hold with the underneath hand to the lower rail, he has better fixation. The lower rail should be approximately 45 cm below the surface of the water.

Underwater lighting

When the patient is in the standing position for lower limb activities, it is much easier for the physiotherapist to observe the movement if there is underwater lighting. It is also much easier for staff and students on the outside of the pool to see clearly what is occurring.

SMALL EQUIPMENT

A good variety of flotation aids is essential and can be of the inflatable type, as well as of materials with buoyant properties such as Plastazote or polystyrene (Fig. 2.2). Also needed are such items as balls, paddles (in the shape of table tennis bats), weighted sandals, Plastazote leg splints and, particularly for children, table tennis balls and a variety of buoyant toys. Floats made of polystyrene should be enclosed in cotton stockinette because, in use, small granules will become detached.

Floats for resistance

A set of graded floats will be required so that progression of resisted exercises may be carried out when strengthening muscle. These can be made out of polystyrene blocks which are easily cut to the required size with even the bluntest of saws. A block of polystyrene 8 cm × 8 cm × 8 cm requires a force of 500 g to submerge it, so that a series of floats should be based on these measurements in order that strengthening in the pool may be related to dry land treatment (Harrison 1980).

Fig. 2.2 Small equipment

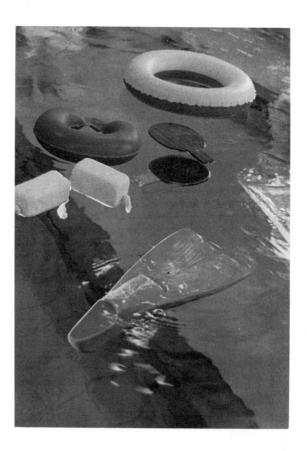

Buoyancy aids

Neck supports

These should be horse-shoe shaped and do not necessarily require straps to keep them in position, although some are provided with Velcro fasteners at the front. The neck supports are inflatable or of Plastazote and are available in different sizes for adults and children. They are invaluable for the comfortable support of the patient in the supine position in the water.

Body supports

It is necessary to have at least two sizes of these. Many departments use old car inner tubes which are inexpensive (or given gratis) and of which there are many sizes. As the valve projects on the inner circumference of the ring, it is important to ensure that it is positioned anteriorly when supporting the patient so that it does not press uncomfortably into his back. Occasionally, due to obesity or some other reason, it is not possible to put a body ring on a patient. An alternative type of support can be provided, made of canvas or stout sheeting with a pocket at each end for a block of polystyrene, cork or Plastazote. Similar supports can also be obtained from commercial companies.

Supports for extremities

A number of smaller inflatable rings in a variety of sizes will be necessary. These can be obtained from toy shops and sport and leisure shops. Preferably these smaller rings should be easily inflatable (by mouth) as the physiotherapist needs to be able to alter the amount of air in the ring depending upon the degree of buoyancy she requires for a particular activity.

Supports for the extremities can also be of Plastazote and with this material it is possible to produce different shapes. When the float is attached to the extremity, the shape of the float will influence the amount of turbulence and, therefore, the drag effect created by the movement of the limb through the water.

Flotation jackets

For many hydrotherapy treatments the float lying position is a common starting position when giving exercises to the lower limbs. Where vigorous movements are part of the programme most physiotherapists find it necessary to add floats to the patient's trunk in order to maintain the position easily whilst the patient concentrates on the exercises in hand.

An inflatable ring around the waist or a pair of floats attached to a sling placed beneath the hips are the commoner ways of providing this additional stability. Flotation jackets have not been particularly favoured by physiotherapists and there are probably a variety of reasons for this, but two main objections have been noted. Some jackets contain blocks of buoyant material which are bulky enough to hinder the movements which the physiotherapist wishes the patient to perform, and this, coupled with the fact that getting the jacket on and off the patient is awkward and time-consuming, provides the reason that most physiotherapists have not considered the use of flotation jackets appropriate to their treatments.

A relatively recent development is a jacket made of bubble film packaging material which is proving popular in a variety of sporting activities and is finding a use among physiotherapists (Fig. 2.3). It is particularly useful for patients with painful backs, for where a ring or sling pulls the back into lordosis the jacket spreads the support and conforms to the patient. At the same time it is loose enough to allow movement.

The average jacket has a buoyant upthrust of about 4.4 kg, and in practice this is about the right amount to support the trunk whilst exercising the lower limbs.

Fig. 2.3 Airlines flotation jacket. (Reproduced with permission from Airlines of Glastonbury, 1986)

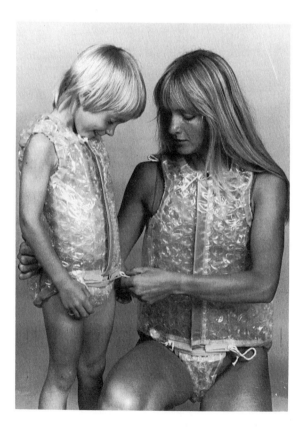

Balls

Plastic inflatable balls can be used in a variety of ways for specific exercises, as well as for games to encourage mobility and for recreational purposes. Table tennis balls are very useful when treating children in the pool and can be used in a number of ways. A range of balls varying from approximately 10 cm in diameter to 30 cm diameter should be available.

Paddles

Table tennis bat-shaped paddles made of perspex or some other similar material are useful in the treatment of upper extremity problems. Two pairs of different sized paddles should be sufficient unless group work is given in the pool.

Flippers

These can be bought in sports shops and are useful for lower extremity exercises and gait activities.

Weighted sandals

Very occasionally a patient with considerable weakness in one or both lower extremities requires assistance to keep the feet on the floor of the pool when doing early standing activities preliminary to gait. A useful aid in such cases is a Plastazote sandal (which can be made in the physiotherapy department) into which is incorporated a weight of a suitable grade (suggested 500 g).

Leg splints

It is useful to have a leg splint (of Plastazote or similar material) available which can be used for patients with particular knee problems. Sometimes it may be necessary, possibly due to pain, to keep the knee joint at rest whilst mobilising and strengthening other joints and muscles. The use of a light plastic splint will enable the patient to work other areas and to do standing and gait activities, but at the same time protect the knee. The knee may also need support in standing and walking if there is a flaccid paralysis of the lower extremity. The amount of support needed in the water is, of course, minimal (p. 122), so that the splint does not need to be as robust as those used on dry land.

SWIMWEAR AND LINEN The amount of swimming costumes, footwear, dressing gowns and towels which will be needed in a hydrotherapy department will, of course, depend upon the numbers of patients and staff, and also upon the frequency and speed of the laundry service.

Bathing costumes

Some patients prefer to use their own costumes and indeed they are expected to do so in some departments. If this is the case, it must be explained to the patient that the chlorination levels maintained in the pool may be higher than those in other swimming pools and that consequently their costumes may show early signs of discoloration and wear. Some costumes will need to be provided for those patients who do not own their own costume or who are unwilling to use it. Patients should be asked to mark their costumes, preferably with a name tape.

The most suitable costumes for patients are those of a stretch material, and they should be one piece as these are usually more acceptable to the patient. For patients with severe disabilities it is, however, a good idea to keep some two-piece costumes. These make changing much easier and quicker, but should only be used with the agreement of the patient as some older women can feel embarrassed when in the pool with other patients.

In a department where costumes are provided, as a rough estimate fifty (total for male and female) will be required in different sizes, usually large, medium and small. Costumes can either be temporarily marked for each patient attending and kept only for that patient, or costumes can be washed through and the patient simply given one from the store each time he attends.

Staff who are working in the pool are often provided with a sum of money from the employing authority for the purchase of a bathing costume. Alternatively, a supply of costumes for staff can be ordered from uniform suppliers or from a sportswear shop, and each staff member loaned a costume for the period during which she works in the pool.

Footwear

Both patients and staff should avoid walking in any area of the hydrotherapy department in bare feet. This will help considerably in preventing the spread of foot infections such as athlete's foot and verrucae (see Ch. 3). Plastic sandals should be provided which should be worn between the changing cubicle and the pool. These should be disinfected at the end of each pool session.

In order to keep the floor of the area surrounding the pool clean, it is the policy in many departments to request all who enter the area to wear plastic overshoes of the type worn in operating theatres. A supply of these placed at an appropriate point will serve as a reminder.

Dressing gowns

Depending upon the geography of the pool department, it is not usually necessary to make a dressing gown available to each patient. In an average department a supply of two dozen will probably be adequate.

Each member of staff will need a dressing gown and these can usually be kept apart and used by the individual for the weeks or months in which she is working in the hydrotherapy department. Dressing gowns should be of cotton towelling so that they can be easily laundered.

Pool 'gowns'

These are sometimes called plombiere sheets, their name recalling their spa origins; they consist of a simple poncho style sheet. They are kept in a hot cupboard in the pool room and are slipped over the patients as they leave the pool. Since they have open sides they present no difficulties when removing bathing costumes and are particularly welcomed by patients who need assistance with this, for whilst preventing them from feeling chilled the gowns also preserve their modesty. For those patients with stiff and painful shoulders it is a relief not to have to manoeuvre their arms into sleeves.

The sheet consists of a large rectangle of cotton material with a centrally placed hole which goes over the head. The dimensions are 2200 mm × 900 mm with a hole of 250 mm diameter in the centre.

Towels

As a clean bath towel or sheet is provided for every patient and member of staff at each attendance, the stock necessary for a department must be calculated taking the following factors into account:
— Expected number of daily patient attendances
— Number of staff in pool each day
— Is there daily collection/delivery of laundry?
— Is there twice daily collection/delivery of laundry?

If there is daily collection and delivery of laundry, it is reasonable to have provision of two towels per patient attendance and per staff member.

Laundry arrangements will vary considerably from hospital to hospital, some having a daily 'top up' service, whilst others will have less frequent deliveries of clean linen. Some departments have solved linen delivery problems by installing an automatic washing machine in the utility room adjacent to the pool and this is attended to by the physiotherapy helper.

Storing for clothing and linen

There should be a properly designed linen cupboard located in the hydrotherapy department, but outside the immediate pool area. In this, all bathing costumes, towels, dressing gowns and footwear are kept. At each laundry delivery, clean linen is unpacked and stored in the cupboard.

In addition to the linen cupboard there should be a hot cupboard in the immediate vicinity of the pool. Towels for the day's pool sessions are taken from the linen cupboard and placed in the hot cupboard and the supply topped up as required. In this way, each patient on exit from the pool can receive a warm towel on his way to the changing cubicle.

STAFFING THE HYDROTHERAPY DEPARTMENT

There is no doubt that the addition of a hydrotherapy pool to a physiotherapy department will require additional personnel. If the pool is sited as an integral part of the physiotherapy department it is usually sufficient to increase staffing levels by two whole time equivalents. If the pool is separate and distant from the main area, more may be necessary.

During a pool session it is reasonable to have two qualified physiotherapists in the pool department and a helper. At least one of the physiotherapists will be in the water with the patients. The helper will be responsible for receiving the patients, allocating changing cubicles, assisting patients as necessary with undressing, escorting patients from cubicle to shower and thence to pool. She will do likewise when the patient has finished his treatment session and assist him in dressing as necessary.

Staffing levels necessary at a pool session will also depend upon the size of the pool (the number of patients who can be treated simultaneously), number of changing cubicles and the presence of students on clinical practice.

In many physiotherapy departments it is usual practice to designate a senior physiotherapist to have responsibility for the day-to-day organisation and supervision of the pool work. It is the senior physiotherapist who is designated safety representative for the area and who must ensure that regular maintenance checks are made of all equipment and who is responsible for the daily testing of chlorine and pH levels. It is not necessarily expected that the senior will be in the pool herself everyday, but that she should control the scheduling of patients and the allocation of tasks to others working in the area. If physiotherapists are working in the hydrotherapy department for some months at a time and are expected to be in the pool each day, it is wise to limit the length of time in water to two hours. This represents, therefore, the treatment time she has available, for the authors do not consider it possible for a therapist to treat patients adequately from outside the pool.

Helpers

In order to ensure the maximum use of physiotherapists' time and skills, it is essential that there is at least one helper allocated to the pool department as long as it is in use each day. In some pool departments helpers go into the pool and work with patients under the supervision of the physiotherapists. Whilst this may occasionally be appropriate, this is not to be encouraged in the pool department in the general hospital, nor in orthopaedic and rehabilitation centres. However, in pools which are also used for recreation and swimming, such as for some children, for the mentally handicapped and for the long term disabled, there is no reason why helpers should not be in the pool with the patients and contribute to the patients' activities under the supervision of the physiotherapist.

REFERRAL FOR HYDROTHERAPY

Pool therapy is just one of the treatment activities available to the physiotherapist, and referrals to the hydrotherapy department must be accorded the same attention and procedure as for those to the ordinary physiotherapy department. Ideally the physiotherapist will have had the opportunity to discuss the patient with the physiotherapist treating him on dry land. If on the other hand the patient has not been seen before, the physiotherapist must examine the patient in the pool department prior to taking him in the water.

A subjective and objective examination is made and the findings recorded. Particular attention is given to the joint ranges and the precise point where pain (if any) occurs. It is also important in the cases of joint condition to discover what amount and type of activity (e.g. whether weight-bearing) produces symptoms in the patient's daily activities. This is because it is so much easier and less painful for the patient to move the joints when in the pool and, therefore, possibly to aggravate an arthritic condition unless the therapist is aware of these particulars. This is explained to the patient, as is the importance for him to note whether there is any increase in pain or stiffness during the hours following the pool session.

When the patient is undressed and ready for the treatment session, he is provided with pool sandals and escorted by the helper to the shower. It must be explained that this is routine and all patients and staff are required to shower before entry into the pool. He is then escorted to the pool, removes his sandals, walks through the footbath and up the steps into the pool. The physiotherapist should be in the pool at the bottom of the steps to receive him. She explains to the patient the different depths, where these change by steps and whether there is a sloping floor to the pool. It is most important to dispel any anxiety or apprehension which the patient may feel and to gain his confidence from the first treatment session.

A short treatment should be given on the first occasion, as it is important neither to fatigue the patient nor to encourage too much activity until it has been possible to assess the effects of treatment.

After leaving the pool escorted by the helper, he again showers before drying and dressing. Following this, the patient is taken to an area outside the pool department where he can rest and have a warm or cold drink. He should be encouraged to rest for at least twenty minutes before leaving the hospital. A few patients who fatigue easily and have a systemic condition may benefit more if, following pool treatment, they are wrapped in a warm towel pack and lie down for twenty minutes. At this point the pack is loosened and one layer removed. The patient rests for a further twenty minutes before dressing and taking a drink.

CHLORINE AND pH LEVELS

The various agents which are used in the chlorination of treatment pools have been described, but the pool manager must understand and be able to carry out the monitoring of the level of chlorine and know what steps to take should chlorine levels stray outside the acceptable limits. Too little chlorine will not have the desired bactericidal effect and too much leads to other problems which will be discussed later.

Monitoring of chlorine levels alone is not sufficient, for an incorrect pH of the water can affect the efficiency of chlorine as a disinfectant and may also have a detrimental effect on the pool plant.

Chlorine

A distinction must be made at the outset between chlorine present in the water which is available for 'attacking' impurities and chlorine which, although in the water, has already combined with other substances and is, therefore, spent. The former is known as Free Residual Chlorine whilst the latter is called Combined Residual Chlorine. The levels of both these types of chlorine are of importance to the physiotherapist and will be monitored regularly.

Free residual chlorine

Chlorine levels are measured in parts of chlorine to a million parts of water or parts per million (ppm). The recommended range for free chlorine is that there should not be less than 1 ppm and not more than 5 ppm. The medium-sized hospital treatment pool is generally maintained at about 2 ppm of chlorine.

Combined residual chlorine

When chlorine combines with organic material in the pool it is no longer effective against bacteria and, indeed, some of the compounds which it forms are themselves undesirable to have in the pool. One such group are 'chloramines'. Chloramines are formed as a result of chlorine combining with nitrogenous material, as is nitrogen trichloride, and these two compounds are said to be the most common cause of a strong chlorine smell coming from a pool. It has been suggested that the commonest nitrogenous substance in swimming pools is urine, and one writer has said that if no one ever urinated in the pool there would be few complaints about pools smelling of chlorine (Humphrey 1978).

As chlorine is added to the pool containing nitrogenous material, chloramines are formed, but with the addition of further chlorine the chloramines suddenly break down and disappear—this is called the 'breakpoint'. In managing the pool, therefore, the aim must not be to keep as high a level of free chlorine as the bathers can tolerate, but to maintain as low a level as is consistent with producing the 'breakpoint' effect. The amount of combined chlorine should never be more than one third of the total chlorine in the pool, i.e. the free chlorine reading should be at least two or three times the reading for combined chlorine.

pH levels

The pH of a substance is a measure of its acidity or alkalinity and is an abbreviation of the words 'potential hydrogen'. A substance which is neither acid or alkaline, i.e. neutral, has a pH of 7, and numbers below this indicate acidity, whilst numbers greater than 7 show a substance to be an alkali. The treatment pool which is maintained at a pH of 7.5–7.6 will give no problems, for it gives a safe margin against the pool becoming too acid and yet is at a level that does not inhibit the action of the chlorine. The limits outside which the pH readings must not be allowed to go are 7.2–8.0.

Testing chlorine levels

The chlorine levels in the pool are measured by using a small device known as a comparator (Fig. 2.4) and (Fig. 2.5). A sample of the pool water is put into a small glass tube and a reagent is added which reacts with the chlorine to produce a colour change in the sample. The depth of colour produced varies with the amount of chlorine present and the comparator is used to determine this.

The first step is to measure the amount of free chlorine in the sample. 10 ml of pool water are put into the comparator sample tube and a tablet of di-ethyl p-phenylene diamine (DPD 1) is added. The tablet dissolves quickly to produce a clear pinkish-red solution if free chlorine is present. If no free chlorine is contained in the water, then the sample will remain colourless. The tube is then slotted into the comparator and held up to the light when it is possible to compare the colour of the sample with a series of coloured 'windows' which can be brought alongside the sample, one by one, by turning the edge of a disc which projects from the side of the comparator. When the sample matches one of the standard colours the free chlorine level is read off directly from figures printed on the edge of the disc (Fig. 2.6).

The total chlorine, i.e. free + combined, is determined by adding a further tablet to the existing solution, but the second tablet is a different reagent DPD 3. If combined chlorine is present the solution will become a darker colour and this is again matched to the appropriate 'window' and the reading noted.

By subtracting the free chlorine from the total chlorine we arrive at a value for the combined chlorine, e.g.:

Reading 1   Sample DPD 1   = 2.0 ppm = Free chlorine
Reading 2   Sample DPD 1 DPD 3 = 2.5 ppm = Total chlorine
Reading 2 − Reading 1   = 0.5 ppm = Combined
                                                   chlorine

As stated earlier, combined chlorine is undesirable in the pool and it is usually recommended that the free chlorine should be two or three times greater than the combined chlorine.

Testing the pH level

Maintenance of a suitable pH has already been mentioned (p. 36), and since some chlorinating agents also affect the pH, it is necessary to monitor it regularly in order that the necessary adjustments may be made promptly. The reagent used is phenol red and this is available in tablet form. The procedure is identical to that used to measure the chlorine levels. The 10 ml sample, with reagent added, is placed in the comparator and colour matched to a different set of standard colours. The pH value is read off the comparator in the same way as the chlorine values after substituting another disc in place of the one used for reading chlorine levels.

Fig. 2.4 Lovibond comparator, front view. (Reproduced with permission from The Tintometer Ltd, Salisbury, 1986)

Fig. 2.5 Lovibond comparator, rear view. (Reproduced with permission from The Tintometer Ltd, Salisbury, 1986)

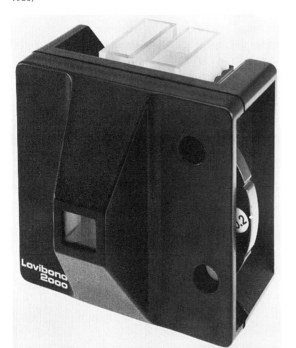

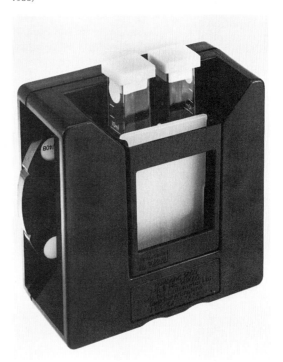

Fig. 2.6 Interchangeable disc for comparator. (Reproduced with permission from The Tintometer Ltd, Salisbury, 1986)

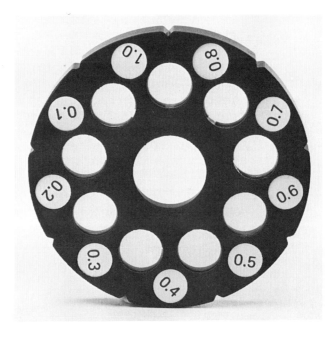

Adjustment of pH

As mentioned previously (p. 38) there is a tendency for sodium hypochlorite to gradually produce an alkaline pool. The reason for this lies in the method of manufacture of the sodium hypochlorite which is produced by passing chlorine gas through caustic soda and some of the caustic soda is left unchanged deliberately because it improves the stability of the bleaching solution.

Large municipal pools introduce acid continuously via a dosing pump to counteract the alkalinity, but this is not usually considered necessary in a small hospital treatment pool. The adjustment is made when necessary by occasional hand dosing with a small quantity of acid. Sodium bisulphate crystals are commonly used and are purchased from pool suppliers as 'dry acid'. The pH of the pool rarely changes rapidly; there is usually a slow trend which one can observe if the pH is monitored daily. Adjustments should be done slowly on a trial and error basis, otherwise over-correction will produce other problems.

Pool capacity

It is necessary for the physiotherapist to know the capacity of the pool in order to estimate the amounts of chemical which may need to be added from time to time.

It may be necessary to 'hand chlorinate' the pool in the event of a failure of the automatic chlorinating apparatus, to bring the chlorine levels up quickly after refilling or to 'shock dose' or hyperchlorinate.

Other chemicals may also need to be added, and the dosage must be calculated from the maker's recommendations and the volume of water to be treated.

In Britain it is still usual to give the volumes of pools in gallons, and the easiest way to do this is to first calculate the volume in cubic feet and to multiply this by 6.25, which is the number of gallons in 1 cubic foot.

For pools with level lanes, one can work out the volume of water represented by each lane and then add these together. When calculating the volume of water in a pool with a regularly sloped base, the depth can be taken at a point halfway along the length:

Volume of pool (gallons) = length (feet) × width (feet) × depth (feet) × 6.25

Calculation of the capacity in litres is rather easier:

Volume (litres) = length (meters) × width (meters) × depth (meters) × 1000

BACTERIOLOGICAL SAMPLING OF POOL WATER

The warm water of the hydrotherapy pool is an ideal environment for many pathogenic and non-pathogenic organisms, hence the need for the scrupulous attention to maintaining the correct levels of disinfecting agent in the water.

With adequate assessment of patients and the taking of suitable precautions the introduction of pathogenic organisms into the pool by patients should not be a problem.

Pseudomonas aeruginosa

This is an organism which will appear in the pool with amazing rapidity after a relatively short period of low values of free available chlorine. Its rapid appearance is probably due to the fact that the pool filter acts as a reservoir, for in the corners of the filter bed where the water is moving slowly or not at all, pseudomonas is able to survive at the relatively low chlorine level. Should the level of chlorine in the circulating water then fall, the organism 'migrates' into the pool and circulating water.

Should this occur, then the chlorine levels should be raised to normal (or a little above), as quickly as possible. In fact, since there is inevitably a time gap of a day or two between the taking of samples and receiving the laboratory reports, the chances are that the problem will already have been solved if chlorine levels have been properly monitored and appropriate action taken. Nevertheless, the physiotherapist in charge should make every effort to find out the reason for the occurrence.

It is this organism which is responsible for swimming pool rash, and this is more likely to occur in the presence of the organism the longer the person is in the water. The reason for this is that swimming pool rash takes the form of a folliculitis and the follicles are more vulnerable when the natural oils are washed away by long periods in the pool.

True swimming pool rash should not be confused with skin irritation which many physiotherapists occasionally get after working in the pool. One must remember that chlorinated water is not a natural environment for the human skin.

Otitis externa can also be caused by *Pseudomonas aeruginosa*, but this would be unlikely in the hydrotherapy pool where underwater swimming would be the exception for most patients.

Coliform organisms

These are the organisms which occur naturally in the human colon and are present in large numbers. Since they cannot multiply in the hydrotherapy pool, if they are discovered to be present, it indicates that there has been contamination of the pool by faecal matter. There is, therefore, the possibility that other organisms which are pathogenic have been introduced from the same source.

This will then call for investigation by the physiotherapist to determine the reason for the contamination. It is when such events occur that the value of carefully kept pool records become apparent.

The finding of *B. coli* should be followed by a few days of higher chlorine levels than normal, but if the contamination is more than minimal it will be necessary to drain the pool. The pool must then be thoroughly cleansed, refilled and hyperchlorinated.

Staphylococcus aureus

This is rarely reported from hydrotherapy pools, but its occurrence will indicate that the pool management is deficient in some aspect and it would be wise to check on the procedures used for monitoring and to seek the advice of the microbiologist.

Taking samples

Samples of pool water should be taken early in the day and it should be arranged that they spend as little time in transit as possible. They should certainly arrive at the laboratory less than six hours after sampling. It is usual to collect the sample directly into a special bottle which will be supplied by the laboratory. The sample should be taken well below the surface of the pool.

The laboratory will require about 25 ml of water and the following information should be sent with the sample if a special form has not been supplied:
1. Place of sampling, e.g. hydrotherapy pool, name of hospital.
2. Date and time of sampling.
3. How the water has been treated: filtered, chlorinated, pH adjusted, etc.
4. Name of person taking sample and to whom the report should be sent.

The frequency with which bacteriological samples should be taken may be the result of local negotiation, but the physiotherapist in charge of the pool should try to ensure that this is done regularly and frequently. It has been suggested that two samples per week should be sufficient.

If it is necessary to take microbiology samples at a time when it is not possible to get them to the laboratory quickly, they may be kept in a refrigerator, but advice should be taken from the laboratory if this is thought to be necessary.

If full records are kept of water treatment and its monitoring, together with the bathing loads, then the additional information from microbiology will provide a useful pool management tool.

Bacteriological 'counts' can appear very quickly, and infrequent random checks of the microbiology will probably miss the possible occasional 'counts' which may be due to easily correctable methods of management.

Hand chlorinating and 'shock dosing'

Most hospital pools will have an automatic system of chlorinating the pool, but some older ones may have to rely on hand chlorination.

In such cases the physiotherapist must first calculate the volume of the pool and then work out the amount of chemicals which must be introduced (p. 40).

There will be times, however, when all pools will need the introduction of chemicals by hand, and the commonest occasion will be when it is thought necessary to hyperchlorinate. This procedure is sometimes called 'shock dosing' and consists of raising the chlorine levels to between three and five times the normal operating levels.

This may be necessary after a high bacteriological count, but is often done as a precautionary measure over periods when the pool will not be used, e.g. bank holidays. It is thought that periodic hyperchlorination will prevent the occurrence of chlorine-resistant organisms.

REFERENCES

Department of the Environment 1985 The treatment and quality of swimming pool water. Her Majesty's Stationery Office, London
Harrison R A 1980 A quantitative approach to strengthening exercises in the hydrotherapy pool. Physiotherapy 66:2
Humphrey W H 1978 Public swimming pool water disinfection. Royal Society of Health Journal 98: 22–24
Penny P T 1983 Swimming pool wheezing. British Medical Journal 287:461
Rycroft R J G, Penny P T 1983 Dermatoses associated with brominated swimming pools. British Medical Journal 287:462

3

Health and safety in the hydrotherapy department

INTRODUCTION

In accordance with the Health and Safety at Work Act (1974), it is the responsibility of all to ensure that the department is a safe and healthy place in which to work. There are many potential hazards to staff and patients within a hydrotherapy department, and a policy which clearly outlines procedures to be followed should be readily available. This must be read and understood by all personnel working in the area. A safety inspection should be made at least every three months by the Safety Supervisor (usually the most senior member of the department staff) and the safety representative. Any faults requiring attention by the engineers or other hospital departments should be reported and rectified as soon as possible.

Hazards in a hydrotherapy department essentially fall into three categories:
1. Accidents
2. Infection
3. Fatigue.

ACCIDENTS

If an accident occurs in the department, an accident or incident form must be completed immediately and copies sent to the appropriate people as stated in District or Hospital policy. A copy of the form should be retained in department files for three years.

Accidents can occur for a number of reasons, e.g. faulty equipment, wet floors, spillage of chemicals (e.g. sodium hypochlorite), incorrect water temperatures, emergency situations and inadequate instructions given to patients.

Equipment

Hoists

As described in Chapter 1, hoists can be operated by mechanical, electrical, hydraulic or pneumatic means. Whichever type is used, the mechanism for raising and lowering the patient must be maintained in good working order. The hoists should be regularly serviced by the manufacturers or by a service engineer on a quarterly contract. Accidents can occur from faults in the raising and lowering mechanism or because the support or chains attached to the seat or stretcher are faulty. It is also possible for the locking and travel mechanism to become defective. Nylon slings (commonly used with electrical hoists) and their means of attachment should be checked daily for signs of wear. Slings should be withdrawn from use if stitching is coming undone or the fabric is rotting due to the effects of chlorine. All staff who may at any time be required to work the hoist, should be given full instructions in the agreed procedure for its safe use.

Submerged plinths and stools

This equipment should be regularly checked to ensure that no screws are loosening and that nylon or canvas slings and straps are sound. Wooden stools or steps should be made of teak or of other similar hard wood and must be checked for signs of splitting or splintering.

Hand rails and parallel bars

Parallel bars are fixtures in some pools, in others they are movable. It is important to demonstrate to the patient the amount of support and stability which can be given by this equipment. Hand rails should be checked to ensure that no loosening of fixation to the wall of the pool is occurring. Grips, handles and rails in other areas of the hydrotherapy department should also be checked to see that they are secure.

Steps

Steps within the pool which provide gradation in depth must be clearly marked by a different or darker colour of tile. The variations in depth must be explained to the patient on entry into the pool. Steps providing access to a raised pool should preferably be covered with non-slip tiles which should not allow 'pooling' of water on the steps. Should the steps be constructed of wood, this should be covered with a ribbed or patterned surface which must be brushed clear of water frequently during a pool session. Checks must be made to ensure that the material remains firmly fixed to the step and does not lift at the corners or edges.

Floor

A wet floor presents a very considerable hazard to patients and every effort must be made to minimise the risks of falls. The floor of both the pool and surrounding area must be surfaced with non-slip tiling. The pool tiles can be less ribbed than those of the surrounding area (for further details see Chapter 1). If water tends to stand on the floor of the pool surround, a stiff-bristled broom or mop should be kept to hand so that surplus water can be swept towards the drain at frequent intervals. Patients should be escorted from changing cubicle to shower and thence to pool entry, and likewise escorted on exit from the pool. They must be cautioned to walk with care, particularly if needing to use sticks or crutches in the area. Although all such walking aids are provided with rubber ferrules, these do not always prevent slipping, which consequently puts the patient at risk.

On leaving the hydrotherapy department wheelchairs must be checked to make sure that the wheels are dry and that no wet tracks are left in the hospital corridor, thus creating a hazard to others.

Care must be taken when providing patients with footwear for use in the pool area. Some patients, by nature of their disability, find it very difficult to walk safely in loose plastic or rubber sandals, and an able-bodied person must accompany them.

On leaving the shower following the pool session, care must be taken to ensure that the patient does not proceed to the changing cubicle with a trailing belt from the dressing gown or a trailing edge of a towel or sheet which could very easily cause the patient to trip and fall.

Chemicals

Sodium hypochlorite

Some hydrotherapy pools have to be chlorinated by hand and, therefore, sodium hypochlorite has to be stored and handled by the physiotherapists. Sodium hypochlorite is a corrosive chemical and should be kept in a cool place and clearly labelled. The dangers in the event of a spillage or splashing of the chemical are to the eyes and skin. Toxic fumes are a danger if a major spillage has occurred in an enclosed area and has been undisturbed for an hour or more. If the chemical splashes into the eye, copious amounts of cold water should be applied, or preferably an eye wash which should be kept in the department in case of this eventuality. If the skin is splashed the area should be flooded with water and any contaminated clothing removed.

Sodium hypochlorite should only be added to the pool when it is empty of patients and staff, and any accidental splashes on the handrails or sides should be wiped off immediately.

Water temperature control

Pool

The temperature of the pool water, which is usually between 35 °C and 37 °C, is maintained by thermostatic control on the plant machinery. If any excessive change in temperature occurs, the engineers must be alerted immediately.

Showers, sprays and douches

All staff and patients must shower before entry into the pool and also immediately after a pool session. The shower should be adjacent to the pool and be large enough to take a patient on a wheelchair and, if possible, a stretcher. Ideally the shower should be in the form of a needle bath (water sprayed from the sides at different levels without an overhead spray), or the shower head should be on a flexible length of hose. The temperature of the water should be 33.5 °C to 35.5 °C and controlled by a mixing valve which has both a manual and thermostatic control. Many patients and staff do not understand the correct way to regulate the water temperature in a shower and it is important that clear instructions are given. In order that both hot and cold water mix in the mixing chamber, the large lever must be fully turned on, the smaller lever is then adjusted to achieve the correct temperature of water being delivered through the spray (see Thermostatic mixing valve, p. 22).

Emergency situations

Cardiac arrest

As hydrotherapy departments are frequently sited at some distance from the main physiotherapy reception area, it is important that staff working in the pool area are specifically instructed in the procedure to be followed should a cardiac arrest occur. It is also vital that certain items of emergency equipment are located in the vicinity of the pool:
— Brooks airway
— Suction apparatus
— Ambu bag
— Oxygen cylinder.
  Depending upon the design of the pool area, a method of removing an unconscious patient from the pool must be practised and all staff working in the area must be familiar with it and in implementing the cardiac arrest procedure.

Drowning

The patient must be immediately removed from the pool, the airway cleared by positioning the patient in the side-lying positions (both sides if necessary) with the head lower than the thorax. Mouth to mouth respiration should be given and the emergency team alerted immediately.

First aid

First aid facilities should be located within the hydrotherapy department to meet such eventualities as cuts and grazes and eye irritation due to chlorine.

All hot pipes, particularly those carrying steam, should be lagged in order that scalds cannot occur. Should a patient or member of staff sustain a scald, the affected area should be immersed in cold water for several minutes. The scalded area is then gently patted dry and covered with a dry dressing.

Alarm system

Every pool should be provided with an alarm system whereby help can be summoned immediately. Staff should be instructed that there should always be a minimum of two able-bodied people in the pool area at any time and all staff who work in the vicinity should know what procedure to follow on hearing the pool alarm. Since the alarm will only be used infrequently it is important that it is tested on a regular basis, not only to make sure that it is functioning, but also to allow staff to become familiar with the sound. The sound of the pool alarm should be quite distinct from other alarms, e.g. fire alarm.

INFECTION

The warm humid atmosphere of a hydrotherapy department renders it an area in which infections are very easily transmitted from one person to another. It is thus essential that all care is taken to minimise these risks. Daily testing of the chlorine and pH levels of the pool water should be done by the physiotherapist, and frequent bacteriological counts should be done by the pathology department or local public health laboratory from samples provided by the physiotherapist in charge (see p. 41).

The chlorine level

This should be between 1 and 5 parts per million, the optimum being 1.5 or 2. The level should be tested before commencement of the pool session and again some two hours later: the greater the number of people in the pool (bathing load), the quicker the chlorine level will drop. The physiotherapist tests the chlorine content of the pool with the aid of a comparator (see p. 38).

The pH level

This should be slightly alkaline between 7.2 and 8.0, preferably in the middle of this range.

The testing apparatus and method is similar to that used to measure the chlorine content, a phenol red tablet being used instead of DPD.1. (see p. 38).

Cleaning

Strict attention must be paid to cleaning all areas of the hydrotherapy department. A solution of 28 g of chloros in 9 litres of water can be used to clean tiled areas including the floor. A stronger solution of 56 g of chloros in 4.5 litres of water is used for gulleys and drains. As these are strong bleaching solutions, protective clothing should be worn and appropriate precautions taken. The deposit which forms at the water line may be wiped off with a cloth dampened with surgical spirit. Physiotherapy aides or porters who clean the pool and pool area should be reminded that chloros or other forms of sodium hypochlorite should never be mixed with other cleaning agents, or chlorine gas may be given off.

Common infections

Tinea pedis

This is a fungal infection of the skin, which is more commonly known as 'athlete's foot'. It most frequently manifests itself by white 'soggy' skin at the web between the fourth and fifth toes usually on one foot only. It very often spreads and affects the spaces between the other toes and may also appear on the other foot. The condition sometimes causes itching at the area affected. In addition, small blisters may appear on the instep which burst leaving a small scaley area. Treatment in the form of local application of an anti-fungal powder or ointment is effective, but spread of the infection to others can occur very easily. In order to minimise risks of infection, patients and staff must be instructed to wear suitable footwear at all times in the pool and changing room areas. Such footwear should be kept for each individual's use and be disinfected in a solution of chlorhexedine at the end of a course of attendances. It is also important that all are educated in the need to dry thoroughly between the toes and if possible to use a prophylactic foot powder after each pool session. Anti-fungal foot powder should always be available for use in staff changing rooms.

Plantar warts (verrucae)

These are found on the sole of the foot and, due to the pressures of weight bearing, grow inwards in the superficial layers of the skin. They are very contagious and can cause considerable discomfort and pain. If during the assessment for hydrotherapy the patient is found to have verrucae, no pool treatment should be given.

Wound infections

No patient who has an infected wound should be treated in the pool. If, in certain circumstances, with the agreement of the refer-ring doctor, the wound can be satisfactorily covered with an oc-clusive dressing such as Opsite, treatment can proceed. However, it would be wiser to treat such a patient at the end of a pool session, thus obviating the risk of affecting other patients. Where it is essential to treat patients with such infections, the Hubbard tank may be used if one is available, since this can be sterilised after treatment.

Acquired Immune Deficiency Syndrome (AIDS)

As the HTLV III virus is transmitted by blood it is essential that patients who are HTLV positive and referred for pool therapy are examined before treatment for any sign of skin abrasions or wounds. If any such lesions are found the patient is not suitable for hydrotherapy. Should an accident occur and the patient bleed for any reason, contaminated equipment (including furniture and floor) should be disinfected with 10 000 ppm sodium hypochlorite. Plastic aprons and gloves should be worn when dealing with this, the items then being disposed of according to hospital policy.

If the patient is treated in the pool, normal levels of chlorination are adequate. (See also page 169.)

FATIGUE

Both staff and patients may become easily fatigued, and general health may be impaired if simple precautions are not taken. Activity and exercise in the warm humid environment of a hydro-therapy department stress the cardiovascular and respiratory systems to a much greater extent than if the activity occurs in the normal physiotherapy department (see Ch. 5). Air temperature in the pool should be 23 °C and humidity no more than 55%. Air temperature in the changing and rest areas should be 20 °C.

Patients

Before a patient undergoes any form of hydrotherapy, the therapist must be aware of the patient's general condition, particularly whether blood pressure and heart rate are normal or within accept-able limits. The duration of any treatment session should be no longer than half an hour. Following a pool session, the patient when dressed should be encouraged to sit in a rest area at a suit-able temperature and have a cup of tea or coffee or alternatively a soft drink. This ensures that adequate time is given for the blood pressure and body temperature to return towards normal and for lost fluids to be replaced. Some patients need to rest more fully and facilities should be available for a patient to rest on a couch in a room adjacent to the department at an appropriate tempera-ture (see p. 67).

Staff

If working in the pool every day, members of staff are not usually required to be in the water for longer than two hours for a maximum of three months. However, individuals will vary in their tolerance to working in the area and heads of department must be vigilant and closely observe staff for signs of excessive fatigue.

This is not a problem which will arise as often as might be imagined, since to some extent staff who seek posts which have a hydrotherapy content are usually those who have worked in the pool and enjoy it. They are, therefore, largely a self-selected group of staff who are not affected untowardly by pool work.

Following a session in the pool, a member of staff should have adequate time provided in which to change, rest and have a drink before resuming duties in another part of the physiotherapy department.

REFERENCES

Atkinson G P, Harrison R A 1981 Safety at Work Act in relation to hydrotherapy departments. Physiotherapy 67: 263–265
Bretherick L (ed) 1981 Hazards in the chemical laboratory, 3rd edn. Royal Society of Chemistry, London
Burton J L 1985 Essentials of dermatology, 2nd edn. Churchill Livingstone, Edinburgh
Chartered Society of Physiotherapy 1979 Policy statements and codes of safe practices. Physiotherapy 65: 17–28
HMSO 1974 Health and Safety at Work Act 1974. HMSO, London
Leppard B J 1980 Tinea pedis. Physiotherapy 66: 48–49
St John Ambulance, St Andrews Ambulance Association, British Red Cross Society 1982 First aid manual

4

Basic physical principles applied to pool exercises

INTRODUCTION

This chapter does not set out to cover all aspects of physics relating to water, for this the reader is recommended to consult a physics textbook. The aim is rather to explain those physical principles, an understanding of which is indispensable to planning a reasoned pool treatment, and to use them to explain the rationale of exercises in water. The progression of exercises in water is quite different in its method to that on dry land, since there are numerous additional factors which must be taken into account due to the different medium. To use dry land techniques in the hydrotherapy pool is to ignore the unique opportunities offered by this medium for the benefit of the patient.

It is not possible to devise a reasoned hydrotherapy programme or to progress pool treatments to suit the patient's needs unless the physiotherapist recognises that a thorough understanding of the basic physics is necessary.

MOVEMENT THROUGH WATER

Since movement in water is the basis of pool therapy, the physical principles which govern this are of prime importance to the physiotherapist. When a floating object is propelled across the surface of the water, it encounters a resistance to its movement, the magnitude of which is partly dependent upon the object's size and partly upon the speed at which it moves. The total resistance has several components, but the two which are of practical importance to the physiotherapist are caused by two familiar phenomena: the bow wave and the wake. The bow wave is responsible for a positive pressure in front of the moving object which is caused by the displaced water, and this tends to impede the object's forward progress. The wake which forms behind the moving object is caused by water flowing into the area immediately to the rear, giving rise to disturbed turbulent water which has the effect of a negative pressure or drag. This tends to hold the object back.

It has been estimated that the bow wave is responsible for only 10% of the resistance and the rest is largely due to turbulence. In fact, there is also some resistance which is due to friction, viscosity and the movement of water at the skin/water interface, but these are minimal when compared to the total resistance.

During treatment the physiotherapist will constantly be required to devise exercises where the resistance is compatible both with the patient's ability and the aims of treatment; this will necessitate varying and progressing the exercises. During free exercise at the surface of the water, adjustment of the resistance can only be made by alteration of one of the three variables upon which resistance depends, i.e. speed, shape and size.

Speed

The faster a movement is carried out, the greater will be the resistance to that movement. If other factors remain constant, then an exercise may be progressed and the muscles strengthened purely by a gradual increase in the speed of performing the exercise.

When a particular exercise, performed at its maximum practical speed, no longer provides sufficient resistance, the physiotherapist must then change one or both of the other two variables, namely shape and size of the moving part.

Size and shape

When we consider the progression of exercises under this heading, we are looking for a way to present the moving part of the body, to the water, in a gradually less streamlined form so that the resistance may be increased incrementally as the patient's needs require it.

Physiotherapists have developed two approaches to this, the first being an alteration of the position of the limb so that the effective lever length, with respect to the muscle group being strengthened, is longer. The second method is to increase the surface area presented to the water by the front of the moving part by the addition of small apparatus.

Alteration of size (lever length)

In Figure 4.1 the patient is seated with the water to shoulder level and the muscles to be strengthened are the shoulder extensors. The elbow is fully flexed so that the surface moving against the water's resistance is represented by the area between shoulder and elbow.

Figure 4.2 represents the same situation, but the patient now has the elbow fully extended. The resistance generated by the movement will now be increased due to not only the greater surface area, but also the greater lever length against which the extensors are working.

Fig. 4.1 Elbow flexed to give short lever length

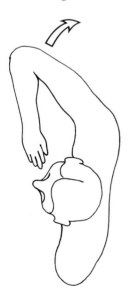

Alteration of shape

In Figure 4.3 the resistance to the same movement has been further increased by requiring the patient to hold a bat which is presented 'face on' to the movement. This radically alters the effective shape of the limb as it moves through the water and results in an increase in the resistance to extension of the shoulder. Obviously, gradation of this resistance between that produced in Figure 4.2 and that in Figure 4.3 may be obtained by using bats of varying size or altering the angle of a single bat so that it cuts through the water more, or less, easily.

Fig. 4.2 Elbow extended to give long lever length

Fig. 4.3 Resistance increased by use of bat

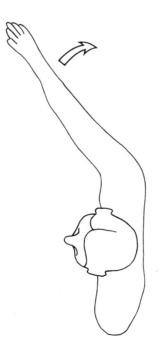

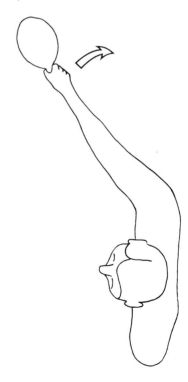

MOMENTS OF FORCE

A moment is a measurement of force which tends to rotate the body upon which it is acting. When a force is applied to an object which has a pivoting point through which the line of force does not pass, then the object will tend to rotate about that point.

The moment of force is defined as the product of the force and the perpendicular distance between the line of action of that force and the fulcrum.

Figure 4.4 represents a man standing in water which comes up to the level of his neck. A float is attached to his hand and the elbow is flexed to a right angle. The moment of force is represented here by the force F (the result of buoyancy acting on the float) × AB which is the perpendicular distance between the line of action of the force and the fulcrum, i.e.

$$\text{Moment of Force} = F \times AB$$

In order to maintain equilibrium, isometric contraction of the elbow extensors must equal this moment of force.

Figure 4.5 represents the same situation, but the elbow is now flexed by about 30 degrees. The force F and its line of action remain unchanged, but the perpendicular distance between the line of action of the force and the fulcrum is now represented by a shorter distance than AB, namely AC. The product therefore of force × distance is less than when the angle at the elbow was a right angle. For the physiotherapist the practical implications in this case would be:

A. Assistance to flexion is at its greatest value when the elbow is flexed to a right angle and diminishes progressively as flexion at the elbow proceeds.

B. Resistance to active extension from full flexion increases as the elbow angle approaches 90 degrees.

Figure 4.6 shows that as movement at the elbow joint passes 90 degrees and extension continues, the resistance to the movement again starts to diminish as the distance AB changes to the shorter distance AD.

The implications of this seem obvious when working out an exercise where floats are to be used as a resistance. What is not immediately obvious, however, is the degree of change in resistance. The variation at different parts of the range of the same movement is greatest where the lever lengths are longest, i.e. where a float is attached to the extremity of an arm or leg. This effect can, on occasion, be an embarrassment rather than a help in cases where a muscle group is very weak or where joint movement is limited and painful, and a seemingly easy movement becomes a forced passive movement. Figures 4.7 and 4.8 show the sort of positions which may give rise to this effect for the knee and hip joints.

In a person of average build and height, the moment of force about the knee joint which is produced by a float attached to the foot will increase by about 4 > × when the knee is flexed from 5

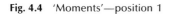

Fig. 4.4 'Moments'—position 1

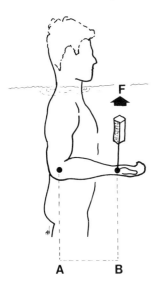

A   B

Fig. 4.5 'Moments'—position 2

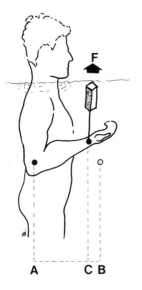

A   C B

degrees to 90 degrees. This is because the perpendicular from the line of action of the force to the fulcrum increases 4 > × whilst the force remains the same. Thus the quadriceps will be required to work four or five times harder to maintain position 2 as they would to maintain position 1.

Because of the longer lever this effect is even greater on the hip joint. On average, the moment of force will increase about six times when the hip is moved to 45 degrees of abduction from 5 degrees of abduction. The adductors of the hip will, therefore, be required to work at least six times harder to maintain a position of 45 degrees of abduction when floats are attached to the foot than they would to hold the leg in 5 degrees of abduction.

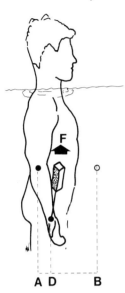

Fig. 4.6 'Moments'—position 3

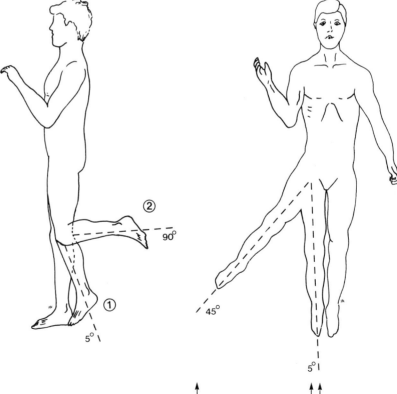

Fig. 4.7 Increase of moment by 90 degrees of flexion at the knee

Fig. 4.8 Increase of moment by 45 degrees of abduction at the hip

DENSITY

The density of an object is a numerical value which indicates the relationship between the mass of the object and its volume. It is represented by the equation

$$\text{Density} = \frac{\text{Mass}}{\text{Volume}}$$

Thus density will always be given as mass per unit volume, e.g. the density of water is 1 g per cc or 62.5 lb per cu ft.

SPECIFIC GRAVITY (SG)

This is an extension of the concept which allows us to compare the densities of substances, one with another, using the density of water as the standard to which the others are compared. For example:

$$\text{The SG of cork} = \frac{\text{Mass of 1 cc of cork}}{\text{Mass of 1 cc of water}} = \frac{0.2 \text{ g}}{1.0 \text{ g}} = 0.2$$

Values given for the specific gravity of the human body are between 0.97 and 0.95. Since the body is composed of many tissues of varying densities in proportions which are different in different individuals, it is obvious that the overall SG of the human body must vary from person to person. It must also take account of the fact that the various parts of the body will have different SGs. The trunk contains the lungs, which reduces its overall SG to well below that of the legs which in consequence will float lower in the water.

To understand fully why two objects may both float, but at different levels, we must next consider Archimedes' principle.

ARCHIMEDES' PRINCIPLE

Archimedes' principle states that:

> When a body is wholly or partially immersed in a fluid, it experiences an upthrust which is equal to the weight of the fluid displaced.

It is this buoyant thrust which accounts for the apparent loss of weight of an object when it is immersed in water or any other fluid.

If, when an object is placed in the hydrotherapy pool, it comes to rest in such a position that its weight is neutralised by the upthrust and a part of the object remains above the surface of the water, then its SG must be less than 1. The proportion of the object which is below the surface would be greater, the nearer the object's SG came to 1. This is because the higher the SG the more water must be displaced before the upthrust is sufficient for equilibrium to be reached.

If, when the whole object is immersed, the upthrust is still less than the object's weight, then it will sink to the bottom showing that the SG is greater than 1.

In the event of an object having a SG equal to that of water, and providing that the object is totally immersed, it will remain at whatever level in the pool it is placed, neither rising to the surface nor sinking to the bottom. All this applies equally to the patient, therapist and pool apparatus and thus the implications are wide ranging and must be borne in mind constantly by the physiotherapist.

It follows from what has been said above that the human body will float at the surface of the pool, but with a large part of its total volume beneath the water line. This may be inappropriate for many treatments and floats are added to the patient so that they float higher in the water. We may think of this as adding appendages to the patient of low SG which result in the patient having a lower overall SG.

CENTRE OF BUOYANCY On dry land we take for granted the effect of gravity and understand the effects, if not the rationale, of its influence. We appreciate that small based objects are unstable and will fall over easily. This is because, for any object, there will be a point within it defined as its centre of gravity. This may be thought of as the point through which a vertical line will pass from the suspension point of the object no matter where this is, provided that the object is suspended freely.

If a vertical line from this point falls within the base of the object when it stands upon a level surface, the object will not fall over. Its relative stability or otherwise will depend upon how close a vertical line through this point comes to the edge of the base of the object. The centre of gravity can be exactly paralleled by the centre of buoyancy.

HYDROSTATIC PRESSURE   At any point below the surface of a liquid, the pressure will be greater than that at the surface by an amount directly dependent upon the depth of that point and the density of the liquid. In water, this is called the hydrostatic pressure and represents the weight of a column of water from the point in question to the surface. This pressure can easily be calculated for any point in a liquid if the vertical depth and the density of the liquid are known. In the hydrotherapy pool, the liquid is water with a density of 1 g/ml and the pressure, therefore, in g/ml will be numerically equal to the depth in centimetres. This can be thought of as representing the weight of a column of water 'standing' on that point.

We must also note that at any point in the water, the pressure will be equal and opposite in all directions. If this were not the case, a fluid could never be at rest since the unequal pressures would cause movement (Fig. 4.9).

Two practical implications of hydrostatic pressure have been noted by hydrotherapists:

1. The effect on distribution of body fluids

It has been suggested that the effect of hydrostatic pressure in the treatment pool is useful in the relief of oedema of the lower extremities and it is interesting to look quantitatively at the pressure involved. A person of average height, standing immersed in water, to neck level, will be subjected to a pressure at mid-calf level of about 120 g/sq cm (1.74 lb/sq in). He is not aware of this increase in pressure on entering the water because the hydrostatic

Fig. 4.9 Pressure in a liquid is equal and opposite in each direction

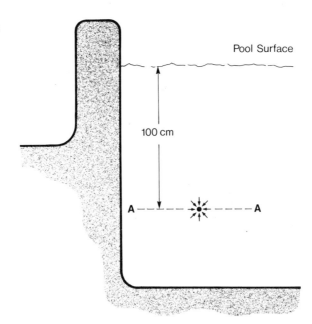

pressure is neutralised by the pressure within the body so that no pressure differential exists across the skin. There is, therefore, no deformation of skin or tissues which would produce a subjective sense of pressure (Neumark 1981) (Fig. 4.10). How does this pressure produced by the water compare with pressures with which we are, perhaps, more familiar?

For example, the pressures beneath a newly applied crêpe bandage on the foot and calf were measured and gave readings equivalent to pressures between 13.5 and 55 g /sq cm (Grant 1983). The pressure on the calf and foot in the hydrotherapy pool is in the order of two to nine times greater than that exercised by a crêpe bandage. The two are not strictly comparable, but even if they were there is still the time factor to be taken into account.

The hydrotherapy session being measured in minutes per week, it seems unlikely the hydrostatic pressure will be responsible for the movement of a significant amount of interstitial fluid during one treatment.

What is more important than the movement of interstitial fluid from the lower extremities is the shift of blood from this region during immersion to the thorax. This is more fully explained in Chapter 5, page 71.

Fig. 4.10 The hydrostatic pressure at every depth is opposed by an equal pressure within the tissues so that no deformation of the skin takes place

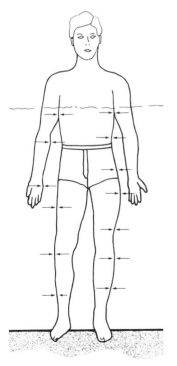

2. Effect on respiration

Physiotherapists have long been conscious that the possible restraint on the mechanics of respiration produced by hydrostatic pressure on the chest wall, could have clinical implications in the treatment of patients with diminished vital capacities. These pressures on an average sized patient would be about 30 g/sq cm acting directly on the lateral chest wall and 40 g/sq cm on the abdominal wall which acts indirectly on the diaphragm.

Besides this small, but sometimes important direct effect there is the indirect effect of the shift of blood to the thorax as already mentioned above. This was shown in a normal subject to be 700 cc (Arborelius 1972). This blood will occupy space normally available for expansion of the lungs and, therefore, results in a decreased vital capacity. Whilst this decrease undoubtedly takes place, its clinical implications should not be exaggerated and a low vital capacity should be an indication to a physiotherapist of possible difficulties rather than a definite contra-indication.

LATENT HEAT

When a solid changes to a liquid, or a liquid to a gas, energy is required to enable the molecules to be separated and to remain separated. This energy must be supplied in the form of heat. Since the reverse is also true, when a gas becomes a liquid, or when a liquid solidifies, that same energy is released in the form of heat as the substance changes its physical state, e.g. when ice is at 0 °C, the heat which is taken up is used solely to change the ice to water, whilst the temperature of the resulting mixture remains the same, i.e. 0 °C. When an ice pack is applied to the skin, the ice begins to melt and the heat required for this is taken from the tissues resulting in their being cooled. This heat, which is required to change the physical state of a substance, but which does not result in a change in temperature, is known as latent heat.

Relative humidity

We are all aware that our physical comfort is dependent not only upon the temperature of our surroundings, but also upon the humidity. This is because the more humid the air, the more difficult it becomes to lose heat from the skin by evaporation of sweat. In all working environments it is, therefore, important to maintain the humidity within the comfortable range. This is particularly important in a hydrotherapy department where too high a level of humidity may easily become a problem. For this reason it is good practice to monitor the temperature and the humidity of the pool room.

The degree of humidity is referred to as the relative humidity (RH). There is a limit to the amount of water vapour which air can hold for any given temperature and when that limit is reached, the air is said to be saturated and the RH is 100%. A sample of air which contains only one half of the water vapour which it could hold will have a RH of 50% and so on. Relative humidity expressed as a percentage is equal to the ratio between the mass of water vapour in a given sample of air and the mass of water vapour it would hold if it were saturated, i.e.

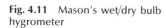

Fig. 4.11 Mason's wet/dry bulb hygrometer

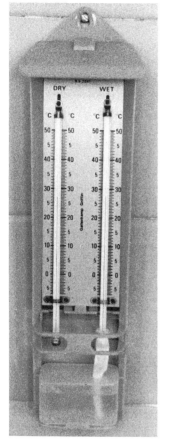

$$\text{R.H.} = \frac{\text{Mass of water vapour in a given sample of air} \times 100}{\text{Mass of water vapour in same volume if it were saturated}}$$

To measure RH directly needs laboratory facilities, but fortunately there is a method of measuring it indirectly which is simple and straightforward. The apparatus used is a Mason's Wet/Dry Bulb Hygrometer which consists of two ordinary, identical thermometers mounted side by side on the same board. The bulb of one thermometer is enclosed in a cotton wick, the other end of which dips into a small container of water (Fig. 4.11).

When water evaporates from the 'wick', cooling takes place locally by the mechanism described under 'Evaporation' (p. 63) and heat is taken from the bulb of the thermometer. This causes the 'wet bulb' thermometer to register a temperature lower than that of the thermometer alongside it.

The difference in temperature readings between the two thermometers will become greater as the rate of evaporation rises and this in turn is dependent upon the humidity of the air. The temperature of the dry bulb and the difference in temperature between the two bulbs are used to read the relative humidity directly from a set of special tables, which are obtainable from Her Majesty's Stationery Office.

For information on recommended levels of humidity and temperature see page 51.

EVAPORATION

Evaporation takes place when molecules 'escape' from the surface of a liquid and this phenomena takes place at all temperatures. The molecules at the surface are in constant motion, but some will have a higher kinetic energy than others, and after leaving the surface of the liquid, they move out of its sphere of attraction and do not return. They then become vapour in the surrounding atmosphere, and thus not only will the mass of the liquid decrease, but the molecules will carry with them their kinetic energy and, therefore, result in a lowering of the temperature of the liquid. For this reason the process of evaporation is always accompanied by a cooling effect on the liquid and its surroundings.

Evaporation and hence its cooling effect are enhanced by a draught passing over the surface of the liquid which prevents accumulation of vapour at the surface, and hence the loss of molecules by the mechanisms described is made easier.

Evaporation is also facilitated by a large surface area of liquid and a surrounding atmosphere with a low concentration of the vapour.

Evaporation and the factors influencing it are of prime importance to physiotherapists, particularly when considering the working environment, and will be discussed later.

REFERENCES

Arborelius M, Balldin U Z, Lilja U I, Lundgren C 1972 Haemodynamic changes in man during immersion with the head above water. Areospace Medicine 43:592
Grant L 1983 Personal communication. Regional Medical Physics Department, R.U.H., Bath
Mills F J, Harding R M 1983 Aviation medicine. British Medical Journal 287:478
Newmark O W 1981 Deformation not pressure is the cause of pressure sores. Care, Science and Practice 1:1

5

Physiological effects and contra-indications to pool therapy

PHYSIOLOGICAL EFFECTS   The physiological responses of the human body to exercise in the hydrotherapy pool are the result of the normal effect of exercise, modified by the body's reaction to an increase in the environmental temperature and pressure. Immersion of the body to the level of the neck, in water of temperature 36 °C, produces marked changes in the circulatory system and the temperature regulating mechanisms but, in the normal healthy individual, these changes take place without untoward effect since the body is well able to cope, at least in the short term, with the alteration in environmental conditions. The normal physiological responses of the circulatory system to heat and to exercise should be familiar to the physiotherapist and will be found in any standard textbook of physiology. What must be considered here is the effect of changes in the immediate environment on those whose physiological responses are impaired by a pathological condition.

One patient, because of his condition, may be unable to make the normal physiological response due to his underlying pathology, whilst to another patient, the normal response may be inappropriate or even detrimental.

Effect on temperature

The human thermo-regulatory system is required to keep the core temperature of the body within very narrow limits and must, therefore, ensure that the heat lost exactly equals the heat produced within the body, together with the heat which may have been absorbed from the environment.

For a given level of heat production by the body, there is a set of environmental conditions which are nearest to the physiological neutral and allow the hypothalamus to regulate the temperature with least intervention. As the environmental conditions move further away from this point the responses will become greater and ultimately a point will be reached where the body will be unable to cope.

The physiological mechanisms for maintaining this equilibrium are:
1. Variation in cutaneous blood supply
2. Sweating
3. Shivering
4. Increase in muscle activity.

The way in which these mechanisms are co-ordinated by the hypothalamus and the inter-relationships of the various components will be known to the physiotherapist. It is important to know, however, to what extent these mechanisms are activated by exercise in the hydrotherapy pool and whether their effects are beneficial or detrimental to the treatment.

Exercises in the warm hydrotherapy pool call for an efficient thermoregulatory system since the body is immersed in water at a temperature of about 36 °C and the natural mechanisms for losing heat, i.e. conduction, convection, radiation and evaporation are rendered either impossible or less effective.

When the body is in air at 35 °C or more, all the heat is lost by the evaporation of sweat, but in the pool at 36 °C, only those parts of the body which are not submerged are capable of losing heat in this way. In addition to the limitation in the body's ability to lose heat, the problem is further compounded by the production of more heat by the exercised muscles.

In spite of the seemingly adverse conditions the normal body is able to meet the extra demands placed upon it by pool therapy when this is given for the usual period of twenty to thirty minutes, assuming that the patient is not debilitated.

It has been shown, however (Fanger 1973), that although there is a wide range of temperature and humidity within which the body can function, the range within which a person feels comfortable is narrow. Fanger was also able to demonstrate that the ambient temperature at which different individuals are comfortable is variable. It follows, therefore, that the temperatures of both the pool and the pool room have to be set at levels which are acceptable to the majority and it is inevitable that there will be individuals who find the pool a little too warm or too cool for their individual preferences.

As a general rule the pool should be at the lowest temperature which is compatible with the comfort of patients and staff, and a difference of only 1 °C will make a noticeable difference in this respect.

Even if we assume that the pool treatment does not have much effect on the core temperature of the body, we must remember that the skin temperature is raised well above the pre-pool temperature. This is one of the reasons why it is usually recommended that the patient be given the chance to cool before dressing and leaving the department (see below).

Some recent work (Barker et al 1986) on serial temperature measurements after pool treatment, has shown that skin temperature of some areas is still above normal long after the usual rest period when the patient rests in the half-lying position. This same study has shown that occasional changes of position seem to initiate and expedite the cooling.

Packing a patient after pool treatment

After most hydrotherapy treatments, and particularly after pool therapy, it is usual to allow the patient to rest before dressing. To this end, it has been traditional to wrap the patient in sheet towels and blankets and to allow him to lie on a bed or couch for about half an hour. One of the reasons usually given for this is that it allows the patient to cool to pre-pool temperature.

If cooling were the prime reason for packing patients, then keeping the patient still, in a reclining position, is probably not the most appropriate way of achieving this (see above). However, in spite of this it still seems reasonable to allow debilitated patients to rest after what can be, for them, a tiring treatment.

Packs of many sorts were used in the different spa establishments and these varied in their complexity. The light pack described here is traditional, simple, but easy to apply and comfortable for the patient. The items required for this pack are:
— 1 pillow
— 2 blankets
— 1 warm full-sized bed sheet
— 1 warm towel.

The bed is prepared by placing upon it the pillow and one of the blankets. The blanket is spread out with its top edge just overlapping the pillow and its edges hanging down over the sides of the bed as in Figure 5.1. The physiotherapist holds the towel in front of the patient whilst he removes his bathing-suit. The patient then takes the top edge of the towel whilst the physiotherapist takes up the sheet as shown in Figure 5.2.

The physiotherapist holds the sheet by its top edge and gathers about a quarter of a meter of it into her hands. The sheet is then placed around the patient's shoulders and crossed over in front of him. The gathered part of the sheet is pulled up over the patient's head as a hood (Fig. 5.3) and the patient is helped onto the couch.

The towel is wrapped around the patient's feet. The top corner of the sheet blanket is pulled diagonally over the patient's shoulder and tucked in; this is repeated with the other corner as in Figure 5.3.

The second blanket is then placed over the patient and tucked in all the way round (Fig. 5.4).

Fig. 5.1 Packing—Bed prepared for patient

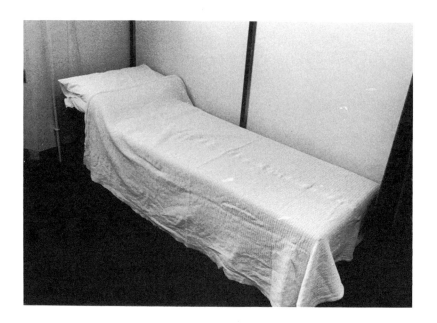

Fig. 5.2 Packing—'Gathering' top edge of sheet

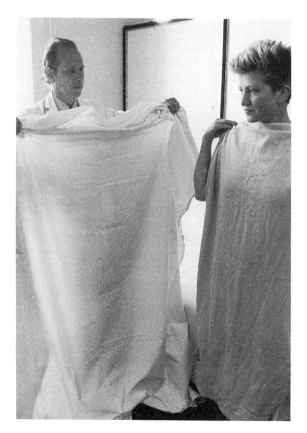

Fig. 5.3 Packing—Applying first blanket

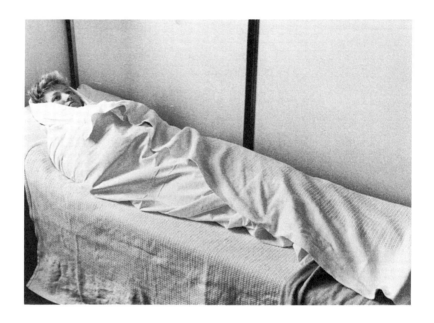

Fig. 5.4 Packing—Completed

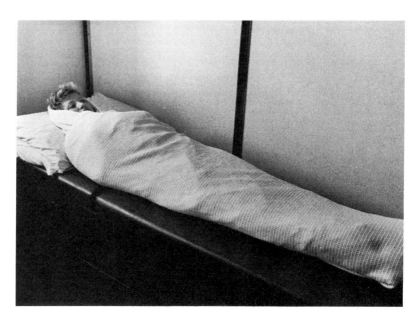

Effect on blood pressure

From the physiological view point, the effect of pool therapy on blood pressure cannot be studied in isolation since it is just one of the results of the inter-related adjustments being made to the circulatory system. As practical physiotherapists, however, it is important to have quantitative data of the changes in blood pressure which may be expected to arise during a typical pool treatment.

The effect of pool therapy on the blood pressure (BP) of 37 patients who attended for a total of 417 pool treatments, has been described by A J Swannell et al (1976). The patients in the study were suffering from various locomotor disorders and all were normotensive or slightly hypertensive. The study showed that there were statistically significant increases in the diastolic pressures as a result of both the pre- and post-treatment showers. There was also a statistically significant drop in the mean BP after entering the pool.

The reason for undertaking the study was to assess whether the changes in BP could constitute a risk to those patients with cardiovascular disease. Four patients exhibited reduced mean BP's below 63 mmHg during treatment and one patient, on one occasion, showed a drop of 44 mm. The authors concluded from their results that the monitoring of BPs of patients with cardiovascular disease was necessary, but that the frequency with which large falls in BP occurred did not suggest that treatment to this group of patients should be withheld.

Acute elevations of BP induced by cooling showers were small and never more than 40 mm and no more than one would expect during normal activities.

Effect on cardiac output

The detailed work on this aspect of immersion which was published by Arborelius (1972) seems to have gone unremarked in the hydrotherapy literature. The work, which was done in connection with space flight, included sophisticated techniques to determine changes in cardiac output and stroke volume when normal subjects were immersed to neck level in water at a neutral temperature. These conditions are, of course, exactly those to which patients are submitted for their hydrotherapy treatment.

It was found that these subjects demonstrated a shift of blood from the legs to the thorax which in turn, produced an increase in the cardiac output of some 30% and an increased stroke volume of 35%. This was presumed to be due to an improved diastolic filling, plus an almost unchanged heart rate.

Arborelius also noted that this was responsible for the occurrence of extra systoles in some of his normal subjects during the first few minutes of immersion. This underlines the possible consequences of pool treatment for patients with cardiac diseases involving coronary insufficiency and cardiac incompetence.

It is worth noting from a practical point of view that the above observations are only valid when the patient is standing in the pool immersed to the neck.

In the supine floating position, one may assume that the mechanical effect of the water is, from the practical point of view, little different to the effect of adopting a supine position on dry land. If the patient is able to tolerate the supine lying position without untoward effect, pool therapy may still be possible if the patient is kept in the supine float lying position.

Renal response to immersion

As has already been mentioned (p. 60), the hydrostatic pressure gradient to which the patient is subjected when standing immersed to neck level in the hydrotherapy pool, results in striking changes in the distribution of the body fluids.

On average, 700 ml of blood moves from the limbs to the thorax (Arborelius et al 1972), and this stimulates the volume receptors which in turn bring about a profound diuresis. The work on this aspect of immersion was carried out on patients with rheumatoid arthritis and normal subjects immersed in water at 35 °C to neck level. Both groups exhibited the same response (Hare et al 1984).

From a practical point of view, this gives a scientific background to the practice of requiring patients to empty their bladders before attending for hydrotherapy.

The same workers found that during immersion a haemodilution occurred indicating that extra-cellular fluid had entered the blood stream. This occurred during the first hour of the immersion and was demonstrated by a fall in the haemoglobin, packed cell volume and red cell count. All these readings returned to normal post-immersion.

It has been suggested that these physiological responses could be important in the modification of disease processes.

CONTRA-INDICATIONS TO POOL THERAPY

Many of the reasons which were formerly thought of as absolute contra-indications to hydrotherapy are now more properly thought of as possible contra-indications. Experienced physiotherapists found that too rigid an adherence to dogmatic rules tended to work to the patient's disadvantage rather than to his advantage (Woodland and Harrison 1983). Over the past few years many physiotherapists have looked more closely at their reasons for ruling out pool therapy and there is now more willingness to judge each case on its merits. This is not to say that the physiotherapist should, at any time, embark upon hydrotherapy treatment if she has any reservations about its safety, but that after assessing the patient, the advantages should be weighed against the disadvantages.

Incontinence of faeces

In most hospital hydrotherapy departments it is not usual to treat patients who have unpredictable faecal incontinence, but in special schools, where mentally handicapped children enjoy hydrotherapy, occasional faecal incontinence may be regarded as unavoidable and accepted as such. In the case of paraplegics where it is possible to evacuate the bowel before treatment, the chances of fouling the pool are virtually nil and this does not present a problem.

Incontinence of urine

This need not be a contra-indication to treatment unless it is suspected that there is a possibility of infected urine contaminating the pool. Catheters may be spigotted, but with the increasing use of condom drainage this is no longer an option for most males. If the bladder is emptied prior to treatment, the considerations are aesthetic rather than clinical since the small amount of urine which may find its way into the pool will be dealt with by the free chlorine and the situation is not really any different to that at any public swimming pool.

Skin conditions and other infections

All infectious and contagious skin diseases are definite contra-indications to pool therapy, although where it is vitally important to give exercises in water it may be acceptable to give exercises in the Hubbard tank if one is available. The tank may then be properly sterilised after treatment, the physiotherapist taking appropriate advice from the microbiologist regarding which sterilising agent is most appropriate.

The infections of tinea pedis and verrucae are considered fully on p. 50. Areas devoid of skin should be covered with a waterproof dressing to prevent infection or cross infection. Adhesive surgical barriers such as 'Opsite' are useful for this purpose and tend to be more reliable than conventional waterproof patches.

The classic waterborne diseases are unlikely to be met in the average hydrotherapy department in the United Kingdom, but typhus, cholera and dysentry etc. are all contra-indications to hydrotherapy.

Psoriasis should not be regarded as a condition rendering a patient unsuitable for pool therapy, unless there are large broken areas which cannot be adequately covered. If the psoriasis is severe and covers large areas, the physiotherapist should be aware that this may give rise to concern among other patients who are attending the same pool session.

It may be necessary to tell such patients that the condition is not an infection and that it is harmless to others. The physiotherapist can always point out that she too is bathing in the same water.

Blood pressure

The stress which immersion places upon the circulatory system and the times during the treatment period when this is at its greatest, have already been outlined on p. 70. Abnormal readings of the blood pressure have occasionally been regarded as contra-indicating treatment, but small variations very rarely give rise to subjective feelings that give cause for concern. High or low readings for blood pressure indicate that care should be taken to observe the patient's reactions, possibly giving shorter treatment times and making sure that the patient has an adequate rest period after treatment.

The heart is certainly required to increase its output during immersion and for this reason it would seem unwise to consider patients with any cardiac incompetence for hydrotherapy.

Vital capacity

Patients with vital capacities which are much reduced from their predicted values based upon age, sex and height should be introduced to the pool with caution. The reason for checking vital capacity and the way in which immersion influences it have been described on p. 61. It is not possible to give actual values for vital capacities below which treatment is contra-indicated. Any values which may be set by individual departments for specific conditions should be stated as percentage decreases in predicted values and not as volumes (Harrison 1981).

Epilepsy

Severe epileptics are not usually treated in hospital hydrotherapy pools, but those whose condition is reasonably well-controlled are treated. When these patients are attending for treatment, all staff who are normally in the pool area should be aware of the possibility that the patient might have a fit and know what procedure has been agreed if this should occur.

Fear of water

There will always be those patients for whom hydrotherapy is the treatment of choice, but who have a fear of water. This may be due to an unfortunate experience in childhood or it may just be fear of the unknown.

With a sympathetic approach and with careful handling on the first attendance most patients will eventually come to enjoy their hydrotherapy. The patients who after a few sessions are still frightened, should not be pressed to carry on with their treatment since little will be achieved if the patient is anxious throughout the treatment.

REFERENCES

Arborelius M, Balldin U Z, Lilja U I, Lundgren C 1972 Haemodynamic changes in man during immersion with the head above water. Aerospace Medicine 43:92

Barker J, Harrison R A, Ring F 1986 Unpublished research. Royal National Hospital for Rheumatic Diseases, Bath

Fanger P O 1973 Assessment of man's thermal comfort in practice. British Journal of Industrial Medicine 30: 313–324

Harrison R A 1981 Tolerance of pool therapy by patients with ankylosing spondylitis with low V.C.'s. Physiotherapy 67:10

O'Hare J P, Heywood A, Dodds P, Corrall R J M, Dieppe P 1984 Water immersion in rheumatoid arthritis. British Journal of Rheumatology 23: 117–118

Swannell A J, Fentem P H, Hughes A O, Trussell E C 1976 Changes in arterial blood pressure in patients undergoing routine pool therapy. Physiotherapy 62:3

Woodland S A, Harrison R A 1983. Re-examination of the contra-indications to hydrotherapy. Tenth International Congress of Rheumatology, Moscow

6

Techniques of exercise in water

When treating a patient in the hydrotherapy pool, the physiotherapist must appreciate that water as a treatment medium has different properties compared with air. Exercise techniques must, therefore, be adapted from those used on dry land, or must be techniques specific in their application to the patient in water.

In relation to the application of exercise techniques, the advantages of the medium of water which are significant in pool therapy are its warmth and its buoyancy, making it a particularly useful treatment medium for certain types of patient.

The human body has a specific gravity of slightly less than 1 and can, therefore, float unaided (see Ch. 4). However, as the specific gravity of the human is so close to 1, the ability to float is critical, and for practical purposes, when active exercise is given in the pool, flotation aids are necessary.

EXERCISE METHODS IN WATER

There are essentially two different ways in which the patient can be treated in the hydrotherapy pool. Treatment can be carried out with the patient supported on a submerged plinth and holding the side of this, or supported in rings and holding onto the rail, or in the standing or sitting position. The method of exercises given with the patient supported in this manner will be described as the conventional method.

Alternatively, the Bad Ragaz or ring method may be used in which the physiotherapist herself provides the fixed point from which the patient works. The patient is supported in flotation rings and does not himself hold onto any fixed equipment.

The characteristics of the strengthening and mobilising exercises which can be given by these two methods differ to some extent. In the conventional method emphasis is usually placed upon exercising one group of muscles in one plane of movement. The rotation component is not easy to assist or resist, although the patient can be encouraged to move to the extremes of range with fixation proximally being provided by the physiotherapist. Patterns of movement are utilised in the Bad Ragaz method and three elements of movement (flexion–extension, abduction–adduction, internal and external rotation) are inherent in all movement patterns, although one or two may be the dominant elements.

Advantages and disadvantages of the two methods

Security

When lying on a submerged plinth or holding onto the pool hand rail supported by rings, the patient feels safe and secure. Any anxieties and fear of water are more easily allayed using this fixation. Supported by rings and floating free, the patient, who is unused to water may well become over-anxious to the extent that little useful exercise can be given using the Bad Ragaz method. However, with understanding, encouragement and correct handling these anxieties can be overcome and the patient can enjoy the freedom from rigid fixation and benefit from freedom of movement.

Comfort

Whilst holding on to the rail or plinth the patient on occasion experiences discomfort, particularly in the neck and shoulder region, and relaxation is difficult. It is easier for the patient who is floating free in rings to relax, providing his head and neck rest on the flotation support.

Manual contact

Although in the conventional method the physiotherapist can give assistance and resistance manually, the method also depends on the use of buoyancy for this purpose. Frequently the physiotherapist is providing extra fixation, for instance at the pelvis. Therefore, it can be appreciated that with relatively little manual contact the physiotherapist does not always have the opportunity to feel the quality of movement throughout range. In the Bad Ragaz method the physiotherapist, by use of her manual contacts and body stance, provides the fixation for the patient in all movements. The physiotherapist who is working dynamically with the patient is thus able to feel and assess the quality of movement and make subtle alterations in resistance through range.

Group work

The use of rings and other buoyant equipment in the conventional method enables the method to be used in treating groups of patients in the pool, requiring only one or two physiotherapists. The advantages of group work can thus be added to that of being able to provide each patient with specific exercises of the required strength, intensity and duration. The Bad Ragaz method can only be used for group work if there is one physiotherapist to each patient, thus it is seldom used.

Staff

As it is not always essential, when using the conventional method, for the physiotherapist to have direct manual contact with the patient, it is possible, if necessary, for the physiotherapist to treat two patients with different conditions and needs simultaneously. Using the Bad Ragaz method the physiotherapist must be on a one-to-one basis with the patient. Thus it can be said that the conventional method of treatment is more economic of treatment in terms of physiotherapist's time, providing that the treatments are equally effective.

Variation

In using the conventional method the physiotherapist is to some extent limited in variation of exercise. Different positions are used depending upon the need for resistance or assistance being given to a particular muscle group; alterations in speed and lever length are used as on dry land, but the method does not provide for easy adaptation to patients' specific problems. However, the firmer fixation of the patient allows the specific techniques of 'hold–relax' and 'contract–relax' to be used.

As the physiotherapist has much greater control of the patient when using the Bad Ragaz method, having direct manual contact, this method provides infinite possibilities of variation of exercise. It is possible to use isotonic and isometric work on different areas of the body at the same time. Specific techniques such as 'rhythmical stabilisation', 'slow reversal', 'repeated contractions', normal timing and timing for emphasis can be easily used. As this method allows for such variation, both patient and physiotherapist working together are well motivated and thus enjoy the pool session.

Size of pool

The size of the pool for use of the conventional method is not of great significance. It is important, however, that there is a hand rail around the pool at water surface level and, if possible, a submerged plinth.

Pool size is important for adequate use of the Bad Ragaz method. The pool should not be smaller than 6 m by 4 m and not deeper than 1 m, except for an area for gait activities. It is possible to use the method in smaller pools, but many of the advantages are lost.

It is important that the physiotherapist working in the pool is familiar with the practice of both these methods in order that the patient receives most benefit from each pool session.

METHOD OF EXERCISES   CONVENTIONAL METHOD

Positioning the patient is a significant factor in the use of this method. The position of the patient will depend upon whether assistive or resistive work is to be given and to which specific muscle group.

The hip

The patient is treated on a submerged plinth with the trunk and pelvis supported, or at the rail of the pool in the corner for easier, more comfortable fixation.

Progression of exercises

Hip extensors

Buoyancy assisting (Fig. 6.1). The patient lies prone and if holding the rail, has the additional support of a large body ring around the pelvis. A small ring is positioned at the ankle of the resting leg for support. The physiotherapist (or patient if he is able) lowers the affected leg to the floor of the pool. She then asks the patient to assist the buoyant upthrust of the water (i.e. actively contracting the hip extensors) to raise the leg to the surface of the water. It is very seldom that the hip extensors are so weak that active movement can only be elicited in this manner and thus in practice this is rarely used. In any case, it is difficult for the physiotherapist to be sure that active work by the hip extensors is taking place.

Buoyancy supporting (Fig. 6.2). For weak muscles, the next progression is more useful. The patient lies on his side with the leg to be worked uppermost. The pelvis and the resting leg, which is in slight flexion and therefore in front of the working leg, are supported as previously. The patient is asked to move the hip through range into extension. It is frequently necessary for the physiotherapist to provide more fixation and she will, therefore, need to hold the pelvis, standing either in front of or behind the patient. If the lower, non-working leg is brought into full hip and knee flexion, this will help to stabilise the pelvis.

Fig. 6.1 Buoyancy assisting left hip extension

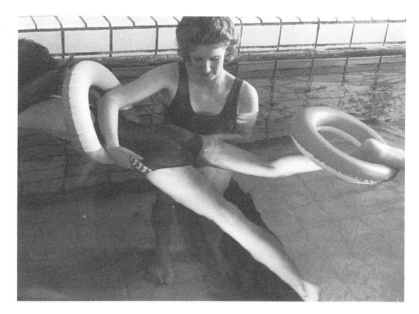

Fig. 6.2 Buoyancy supporting left hip extension, fixation at pelvis by physiotherapist

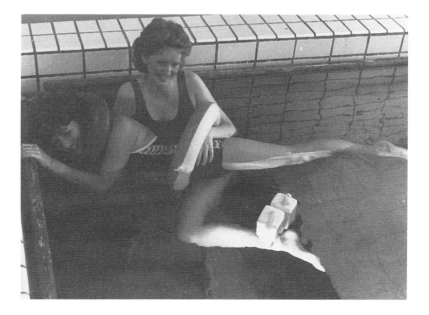

Buoyancy resisting (Fig. 6.3). The patient lies supine, again supported at pelvis and at the resting leg. The patient is asked to extend the hip, moving the leg downwards towards the floor of the pool. The upthrust of the water offers the most resistance in the outer part of range, that is at the nearest to the horizontal (see Ch. 4). To add more resistance to the movement a ring in which there is only a small amount of air can be positioned on the limb at the ankle. The patient must now work against the increased upthrust exerted on the limb. Resistance can be further increased by adding more air to the ring. As the patient is able to work more strongly he requires more fixation in order to ensure that extension at the hip is occurring and not excessive extension of the lumbar spine.

Hip abductors

Buoyancy assisting. The patient is supported in side-lying, the working leg uppermost. The patient lowers the resting leg in the water and the physiotherapist can fix the foot on the floor of the pool by using her own foot. The upper leg is lowered and the patient then asked to raise the leg with the help of the upthrust. As with buoyancy assisted hip extension this grade of work is seldom required.

Buoyancy supporting. The patient lies in the supine position supported at the pelvis if necessary with small buoyant supports at both ankles. The patient either abducts both legs, or the physiotherapist can stand at one side and stabilise the pelvis and the leg on that side whilst the patient moves the other leg through range.

Buoyancy resisting (Fig. 6.4). The patient is again in side-lying with the resting leg uppermost. This can be supported in a ring placed at the ankle. The patient, using the abductors, moves his lower leg downwards towards the floor of the pool. To increase the resistance to the movement, a ring with the requisite amount of air can be placed around the ankle. Extra fixation at the pelvis will need to be provided by the physiotherapist as the patient is able to work more strongly and greater resistances are used.

Fig. 6.3 Buoyancy resisting right hip extension, added resistance by inflatable ring at the ankle

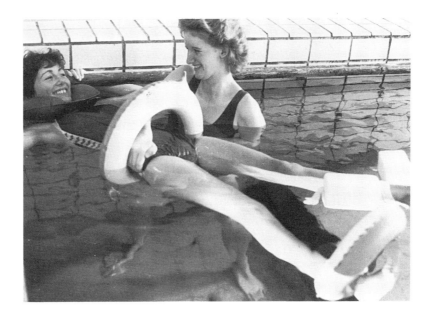

Fig. 6.4 Buoyancy resisting right leg abduction, fixation at pelvis

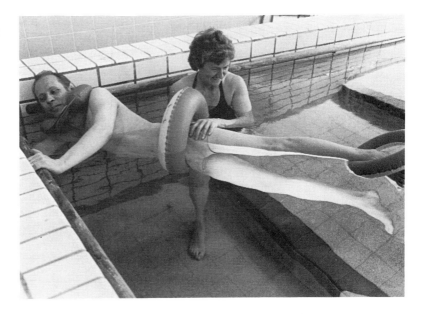

The knee

The patient is treated in the lying, sitting or standing position.

Progression of exercises

Knee extensors

Buoyancy assisting. The patient sits on a submerged stool. In order for the upthrust of the water to exert an assistive effect on the knee extensors, the physiotherapist must assist the initial part of the movement to bring the angle of the knee joint to just over 90 degrees. The patient endeavours to straighten the knee with the assistance of the upthrust. Maximum effect occurs in inner range. The patient can also work supported in the supine-lying position. The hip remains extended and the knee is flexed to 90 degrees. It is sometimes preferable to use this starting position as no tension is put on the hamstrings.

Buoyancy supporting (Fig. 6.5). The patient lies in the side-lying position, supported as necessary with the working leg uppermost. The patient extends the knee through full range, the physiotherapist stabilising the thigh if necessary.

Buoyancy resisting (Fig. 6.6). This can best be done with the patient standing holding onto the rail. He flexes the working knee, the hip remaining in the neutral position. The patient then extends the knee, bringing the foot to the floor of the pool. Although knee extension is occurring against the upthrust of the water, the lever is short and, therefore, the resistance of no great magnitude. To provide adequate resistance to the knee extensors it is necessary to attach a ring or other buoyant appliance to the ankle.

Knee flexors

Buoyancy assisting (Fig. 6.7). The patient stands holding onto the rail. With her foot the physiotherapist assists the patient to move his foot from the floor of the pool. The patient flexes his knee with assistance from the upthrust, the hip remaining in the neutral position.

Buoyancy supporting. The position is as for buoyancy supporting knee extension.

Buoyancy resisting. The patient sits on a submerged stool with the knee extended. He then flexes the knee against the resistance of the upthrust to 90 degrees. Increased resistance is given by the use of a ring attached around the ankle. An alternative position that can be used is supine-lying. The hip is maintained in the neutral position and the patient flexes his knee to 90 degrees.

Fig. 6.5 Buoyancy supporting left knee extension

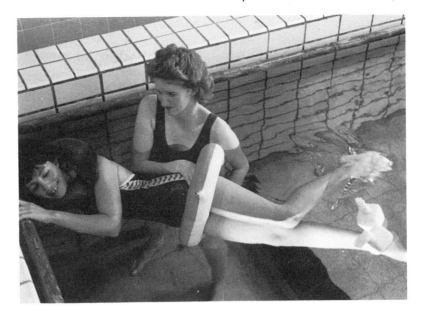

Fig. 6.6 Buoyancy resisting left knee extension, with added resistance from a polystyrene float

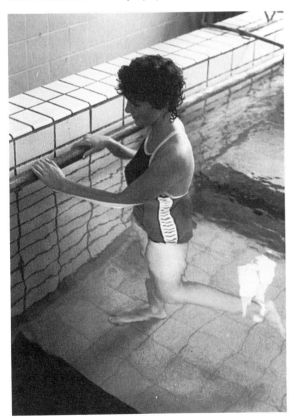

Fig. 6.7 Buoyancy assisting left knee flexion

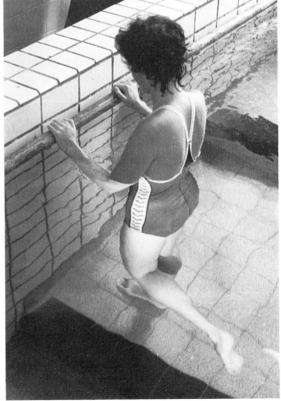

The shoulder

The patient may be treated in a number of positions which will be determined by the type of work required, i.e. assisted or resisted, the plane in which the movement is to occur and the part of range to be emphasised.

Fig. 6.8 Buoyancy assisting left shoulder abduction

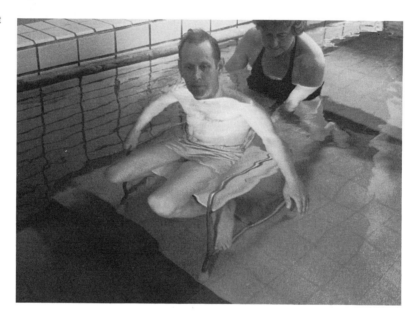

Fig. 6.9 Buoyancy supporting right shoulder abduction

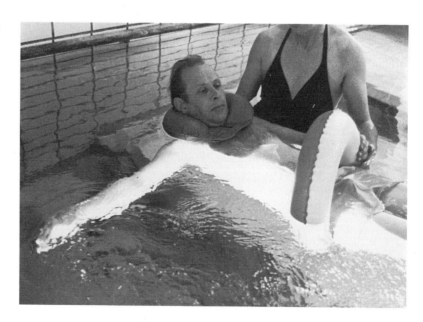

Shoulder abductors

Buoyancy assisting (Fig. 6.8). The patient sits on a submerged stool, the water level just covering the shoulder region. With assistance from the physiotherapist to initiate the movement, the arm is taken away from the patient's side and is raised to surface level, moving through 90 degrees of abduction. If the patient leans his upper trunk towards the working side, a few more degrees of assisted abduction can be obtained. There is no position which satisfactorily allows for buoyancy to assist the inner range of abduction to elevation.

Buoyancy supporting (Fig. 6.9). The patient lies supine supported on a submerged plinth or in rings. It is preferable that he fixes himself by holding on to the rail or side of the plinth with the other hand. Alternatively, if floating free away from the rail, the physiotherapist can stabilise the patient's pelvis. The patient is able to move his arm from his side through the full range of abduction to elevation.

Buoyancy resisting (Fig. 6.10). The patient is in side-lying supported by rings and with additional fixation provided by the physiotherapist: a submerged plinth cannot be used. The working arm is underneath, resting against the patient's side. Resistance to abduction is given by the upthrust as the patient moves the arm downwards in the water to 90 degrees abduction. Further resistance is given if the patient holds a ring or buoyant float.

Fig. 6.10 Buoyancy resisting right shoulder abduction, with added resistance of a polystyrene float held in the patient's hand

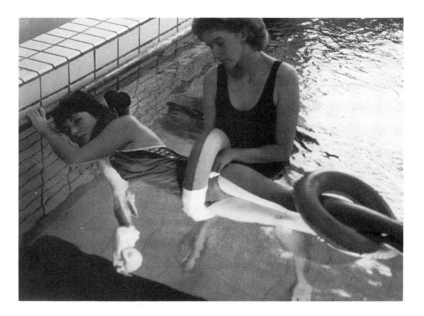

Shoulder flexors

Buoyancy assisting (Fig. 6.11). The patient is in sitting, and as with the exercise using buoyancy to assist shoulder abduction, the physiotherapist initiates the flexion movement so that buoyancy can assist the patient's efforts to flex the shoulder, the arm being raised to surface level.

Buoyancy supporting. In the side-lying position the patient lies supported on a plinth or in rings, the working arm uppermost. The arm can be moved through full range, the physiotherapist fixing the trunk as necessary.

Buoyancy resisting. This is difficult to achieve satisfactorily, and alternative means of resisting shoulder flexion will be described later in the chapter. Buoyancy can be used to provide resistance if the patient can lie in the prone position supported by rings. The arm is moved from the patient's side downwards to reach an angle of 90 degrees. Additional resistance can be given by the use of an extra ring or float which the patient holds.

The foregoing section provides examples of the ways in which buoyancy can be used to assist or resist a movement and to provide progression in strengthening a muscle group. The principles can be applied to any muscle group in the body, but those described are the most frequently used. It is difficult to use buoyancy to assist or resist the rotator muscles around a joint. Rotation can be added to the movement, for instance hip extension, buoyancy resisting, by asking the patient as he pushes the leg downwards, to turn the heel out, so working the medial rotators of the hip. However, resistance cannot be given to the rotation component except manually, and this is perhaps one of the disadvantages of this method.

When adding further resistance to a buoyancy resisted movement by using an additional ring, it must be clearly explained to the patient that the limb must return to the starting position in a controlled manner. Eccentric muscle work is required, and it is important that the physiotherapist ensures that the patient has sufficient muscle power to prevent an uncontrolled movement. This is particularly important in painful joint conditions such as rheumatoid arthritis, or when the patient has undergone joint replacement surgery.

By using specially made floats for resisted exercises, it is possible to grade strengthening exercises quantitatively so that they may be compared directly with those on dry land. Polystyrene packing material is a conveniently available material for making such floats and if these are made in units of 8 cm cubes, the physiotherapist will have a means of increasing resistances by increments of 500 g (Harrison 1980).

Further means of altering the resistance

As well as the use of buoyancy, other physical principles can be applied to increase or decrease the resistance offered to a movement. The speed at which the movement is performed, and the size and shape of the limb or moving part of the body, are three variables upon which resistance depends (see Ch. 4). In practice, it is more usual to increase the speed of the movement and to increase the turbulence (drag effect) than to lengthen the lever to provide greater resistance.

It must always be remembered that when a limb moves in a vertical plane from the surface of the water towards the floor of the pool or vice versa, the effect of buoyancy on the movement will be reversed if the limb moves through more than 90 degrees.

Fig. 6.11 Buoyancy assisting right shoulder flexion

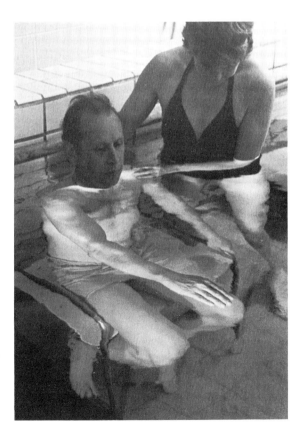

The trunk

Firm fixation is required for trunk exercises and can be given at the upper extremities and upper trunk, or alternatively at the lower extremities or pelvis. Use of the hand rail or sides of the submerged plinth provides easy and firm fixation.

Trunk side flexors

Buoyancy assisting. The patient is in side-lying holding firmly on to the hand rail. The physiotherapist stands behind the patient and adds fixation at the lower thorax. The patient is in trunk side flexion with both feet resting on the floor of the pool. The physiotherapist assists in initiation of the movement by moving the feet from the floor of the pool. The patient attempts to work the trunk muscles of the side uppermost as the upthrust assists the movement.

Buoyancy supporting (Fig. 6.12). Lying, supported in rings or on the submerged plinth, the patient holds on to fixed rails with both hands. A ring is passed around both ankles so that the legs are held together. Full range side flexion to the right and left can be achieved as the legs and lower trunk are moved to each side with the upper trunk and arms fixed. Alternatively the patient, supported in rings, puts his toes under the hand rail so that fixation is distal (feet slightly apart), the upper trunk is then moved from side to side through full range.

Buoyancy resisting (Fig. 6.13). The patient is in side-lying, supported in rings and holding the hand rail. The patient moves both legs together downwards towards the floor of the pool against the upthrust. Additional rings can be placed around the legs to provide more resistance.

Fig. 6.12 Buoyancy supporting trunk right side flexion

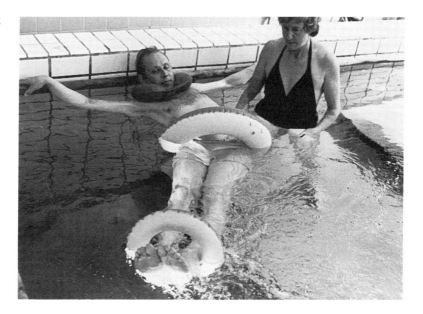

Fig. 6.13 Buoyancy resisting trunk right side flexion

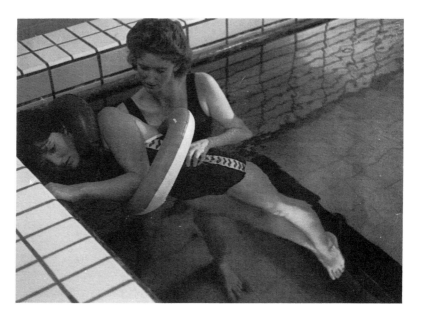

Trunk extensors

Buoyancy assisting. The patient lies in the prone position with a ring supporting high in the abdominal region; he holds a hand rail for fixation, both feet are on the floor of the pool. The physiotherapist assists in the initiation of the movement as buoyancy assists the raising of the legs and lower trunk, the patient also working as far as possible through range.

Buoyancy supporting. In side-lying, supported in rings, fixation can be provided either by the patient holding the hand rail or with the physiotherapist holding around the patient's pelvis. Full range trunk extension is possible in this position.

Buoyancy resisting (Fig. 6.14). The patient lies in supine holding the hand rail. A body ring supporting the upper trunk or additional manual fixation by the physiotherapist will prevent excessive movement occurring at the shoulder region. The patient pushes both legs which are held together downwards in the water. Resistance can be increased by the use of a ring around the ankles.

Trunk flexors

The starting positions for buoyancy assisted and buoyancy resisted trunk flexion are the reverse of those for trunk extension. Buoyancy supporting exercises are given in the same position as for trunk extension.

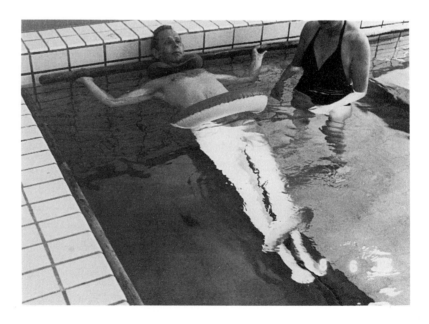

Fig. 6.14 Buoyancy resisting trunk extension

THE BAD RAGAZ OR RING METHOD

This method of exercise in water has been developed in Bad Ragaz, Switzerland and is now widely used in many countries. In this method, buoyancy is used in its supportive function and not as a means of providing resistance. The patient is not required to hold the rail nor does he need the support of a submerged plinth.

The physiotherapist provides the fixation for the patient and she must, therefore, be in the water and work on a one to-one basis with the patient, throughout the treatment sessions.

Resistance to a movement is provided by the movement of the body through the water causing turbulence which results in a drag or 'negative' force which opposes the movement and by the bow wave (10% approximately). Resistance is increased by faster movement of the body through the water, by altering the shape of the limb (addition of floats, rings, etc.), by distal fixation, and by the physiotherapist moving in the direction of the movement as she provides the fixation.

As a form of resisted exercise the Bad Ragaz method is unique in that the resistance is self-regulating. In other methods, provision of the maximum resistance required for muscle strengthening must be adjusted by the physiotherapist.

In the Bad Ragaz method the resistance increases as the speed of the movement increases, and providing the patient is working to his maximum, the speed and thus the resistance will adjust itself to the patients' capabilities.

Resistance can be decreased by reducing the speed of movement, by the use of more proximal holds (shortening the lever) and by the physiotherapist moving the fixation she provides in the opposite direction to the movement.

Use of this method of exercise in water enables the physiotherapist to work muscles and joints in patterns of movement, rather than isolating activity to one group of muscles or to one joint, and to use the principles of proprioceptive neuromuscular facilitation. However, if only one joint is to be moved, the techniques used in this method can be adapted to this purpose, and at the same time the whole muscle synergy can be activated in the normal sequence.

Similarly, if there is weakness in some of the muscles in the movement pattern, the stronger muscles can be used to irradiate into the weaker ones, or alternatively, stronger muscles of the contra- lateral limb or trunk can be used for irradiation of activity. Isometric work can be given, and in particular the postural stabilising function of any muscle group can be exercised. Specific techniques such as repeated contractions, slow reversals, quick stretch and rhythmical stabilisation can be used to good advantage. The rotation component of all muscle groups can be resisted or assisted, ensuring maximum response to the demand placed upon the muscle action.

Most patterns are worked with the patient in supine-lying, supported by a body ring in the lower lumbar or pelvic area; a neck float and other small rings are used as necessary. Some trunk patterns are best done in side-lying, and to work the flexion and extension components of the shoulder effectively the patient is treated in the prone position.

As the patient is not able to hold the rail when these techniques are being used, it is extremely important that the physiotherapist provides sufficient stability and fixation for the patient. A patient on his first attendance may be apprehensive and anxious that any movement he is asked to make will result in instability and a fear of capsizing.

The human body, when floating and supported by rings, can be said to be in a state of stable equilibrium, although this is only true of a body which is symmetrical in form in its presentation to the water. For example, absence of a limb or part of a limb, spasticity or contracture of a limb or trunk or a rotational deformity of head, trunk or limbs will have the effect of making the body asymmetrical and, therefore, less stable in water.

It is very easy during treatment to disrupt the equilibrium, even though the use of flotation aids do assist in the stability of the patient in water. The physiotherapist must be aware of this tendency and handle the patient appropriately. When one limb is flexed during a movement there is a tendency for the patient to roll towards that side as there is less body surface in the water on which the upthrust has an effect, and more body surface presenting on the contra-lateral side. The patient can counteract this by turning his head away from that side, or he can rest the contra-lateral arm on the body ring. However, in practice these moves are seldom necessary as the flotation aids (neck support and body ring) aid the stability, and with experienced handling by the physiotherapist rolling can be prevented.

Proximal and distal holds

In using this technique, the physiotherapist's hands are positioned on the limbs or trunk in a number of ways. Positioning of her hands will influence the movement of the patient, the emphasis to be placed on certain muscle groups and the amount of isometric or isotonic work required. Positioning of the physiotherapist's hands can also assist in the ease of handling the patient, as well as providing more stability for the patient during exercises in the water. If a patient is severely disabled, has gross flaccid paralysis, or is particularly anxious in the water, the physiotherapist will find it easier to handle the patient if she uses proximal hand holds. The anxious patient will also feel more controlled and safer with proximal fixation by the physiotherapist. To provide maximum control, the most proximal holds at thorax and pelvis should be used with the patient in the supine position.

Moving slightly more distally, the mid-thigh region, below the knee around the tibia, and, more distally, the foot and finally the toes are the most usual points of fixation. Manual holds of the upper extremity can also be varied as for the lower extremity.

It should be realised that by moving the hand holds more distally, more muscle work is demanded of the patient, and this in itself is a means of increasing resistance to exercise in terms of the demand placed upon the cardiovascular and respiratory systems.

Some examples of the ways in which this technique can be used are given in the following pages. The patterns described are those most commonly used, but it will be realised that this technique offers enormous flexibility. The individual physiotherapist will develop ways in which she can use the principles to the advantage of the patient she is treating. Different patterns of movement will be used depending upon the muscle groups to be strengthened or joint range increased. If required, rolling and correcting a tendency to roll, can be useful activities.

The resistances which are produced by the various patterns will have limits beyond which they cannot be increased, and if at this point the muscle needs further strengthening other methods must be used.

The limit for a particular pattern will be reached at the maximum speed with the most distal hand holds, and the quantitative value will vary from pattern to pattern.

In general, it has been shown (Harrison and Alland 1982) that patterns of Ab and adduction approach full resistance to normal muscles, whilst those of flexion and extension do not.

Lower extremity patterns

Left leg, hip extension, abduction and medial rotation, knee extension, plantar flexion with eversion (Figs 6.15 and 6.16)

The patient lies in the supine position, supported by rings at neck and pelvis; a small ring can be placed around the ankle of the right leg, the left is in flexion, adduction and lateral rotation, the knee flexed and the foot dorsi-flexed and inverted. The physiotherapist stands in the walk–stand position close to the patient's left foot, slightly to the side. One hand is placed on the plantar surface of the foot, the other on the posterior aspect of the thigh (to emphasise the hip activity), or under the knee to better resist and guide the rotation component and to prevent excessive extension at the knee if this would be painful. The patient is asked to turn the knee in and push the foot down and out; as he extends the leg he moves through the water away from the physiotherapist. The hip extends, abducts and medially rotates, the knee extends and the foot plantar flexes and everts. The physiotherapist leans forward into the movement, keeping the fixation point of the foot close to her side. She resists (or assists) the muscle work, guiding the leg through the pattern and resisting (or assisting) all three components of the movement. At the extent of the movement the patient is asked to relax, the physiotherapist walking forwards as she flexes the leg to regain the starting position.

Fig. 6.15 Starting position for left hip extension, abduction, medial rotation, knee extension, plantar flexion with eversion

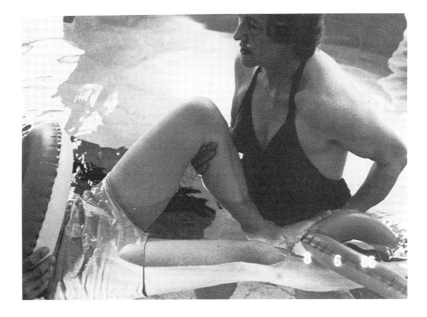

Fig. 6.16 End of range for left hip extension, abduction and medial rotation pattern

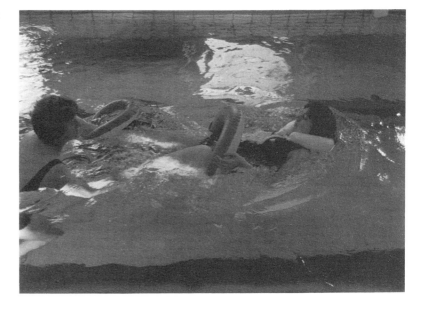

Left leg, hip flexion, adduction, lateral rotation, knee flexion, dorsiflexion with inversion (Figs. 6.17 and 6.18)

The patient is in the supine supported lying position, the leg extended, abducted and medially rotated at the hip. The physiotherapist stands at the left foot of the patient, placing the left hand on the dorsum of the patient's left foot. The physiotherapist's other hand is placed more proximally where required, usually on the antero-medial aspect of the thigh. The patient is asked to pull the foot up and bend the leg. The physiotherapist again resists or assists and guides the movement, this time leaning and stepping backwards as the patient comes towards her, that is, always in the direction of the movement. The patient relaxes, the leg is extended and the movement repeated.

In order to resist more strongly or assist the abduction/adduction component, it is easier to do so with a bilateral pattern and straight knees.

Fig. 6.17 Starting position for left hip flexion, adduction, lateral rotation, knee flexion, dorsi flexion with inversion

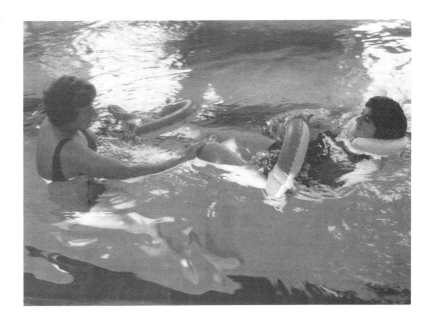

Fig. 6.18 End of range for left hip flexion, adduction, lateral rotation pattern

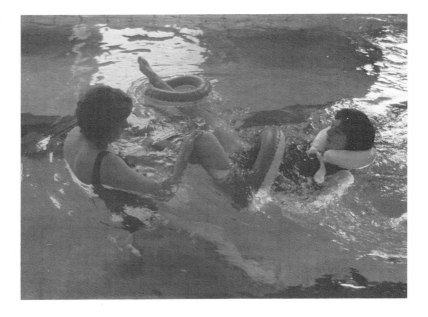

Fig. 6.19 Mid-range bilateral hip extension, abduction and medial rotation

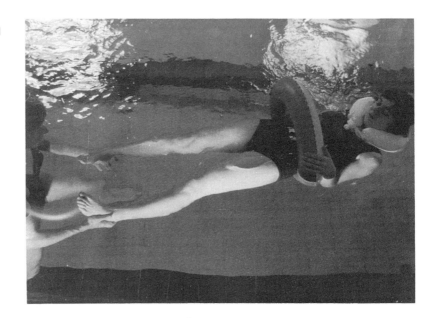

Fig. 6.20 End of range bilateral hip extension, abduction and medial rotation

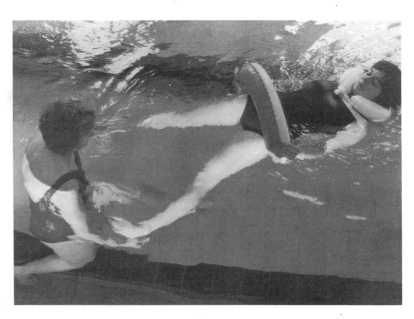

Bilateral hip extension, abduction and medial rotation (Figs 6.19 and 6.20)

The physiotherapist stands at the patient's feet in the walk—standing position. She places a hand on the postero-lateral aspect of each heel, the patient again in the supported supine-lying position, with legs together, knees extended and hips laterally rotated. The patient is asked to push both heels down and out, the physiotherapist resisting the movement and moving her hands downwards and sideways, leaning backwards as the patient moves through the water towards her.

Bilateral hip extension, adduction and lateral rotation (Fig. 6.21)

Hip adduction is better emphasised with extension of the hip rather than in a flexion pattern. The patient is in the supported supine position, the physiotherapist standing at his feet. The physiotherapist places her hands on the postero-medial aspect of the patient's heels, the knees being straight with hips abducted, medially rotated and slightly flexed so that the heels are just out of the water. The patient is asked to bring the heels down and together; as he does so the physiotherapist resists and guides the patient through the movement as he moves away from her. The physiotherapist leans into the movement and takes a step forwards as the patient moves through the water.

Fig. 6.21 Mid-range bilateral hip extension, adduction and lateral rotation

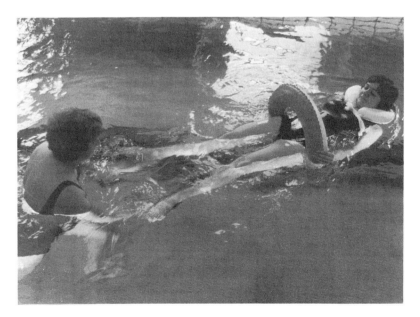

Right leg hip extension, abduction and medial rotation, to emphasise the abduction component (Fig. 6.22)

The patient is in supine supported in rings; the physiotherapist stands at the patient's left side, facing to the right. She places her right hand on the left lateral aspect of the pelvis and her left hand on the lateral aspect of the left leg at the ankle or heel. The patient is asked to push the right leg sideways, turning the heel downwards and outwards as he does so. The physiotherapist leans into the movement, giving firmer fixation at the ankle than at the pelvis. At the end of range the patient relaxes, the physiotherapist brings the left leg to the right leg, and the movement is repeated. The movement occurs through the arc of a circle, the bow wave and turbulence being caused chiefly by the movement of the right leg through the water. The muscle work at the right hip is isotonic and the leg moves dynamically, but activity in the left leg is not entirely isometric. As the right hip moves towards the end of range, there is effective abduction occurring in the left hip as the pelvis tilts.

There is an alternative method for the physiotherapist to provide fixation for this movement and to increase the stabilising activity of the trunk muscles on the left. The physiotherapist holds the patient's left hand in her right hand. The fixation on the lateral aspect at the ankle remains as previously. The patient, keeping the elbow straight, extends, abducts and medially rotates at the shoulder; the physiotherapist resists the activity and a static hold is built up and maintained working latissimus dorsi whilst the right leg is moving through range.

Right leg, extension, adduction lateral rotation, to emphasise the adduction component (Fig. 6.23)

This pattern is the reverse of the above movement. The physiotherapist places her left hand on the medial aspect of the left ankle, her right hand is placed on the medial aspect of the left upper thigh, the legs are abducted. The patient is asked to bring the right leg to the left, turning the heel in and slightly downwards, the physiotherapist leans backwards as the right leg is adducted to the left leg. The arc of a circle is again described.

Fig. 6.22 Single leg (right) hip extension, abduction and medial rotation. Note physiotherapist leaning into the movement

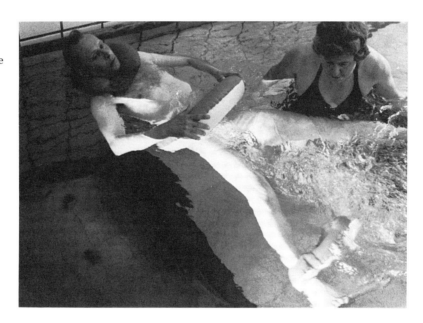

Fig. 6.23 Single leg (right) hip extension, adduction and lateral rotation. Physiotherapist leaning backwards in the direction of movement

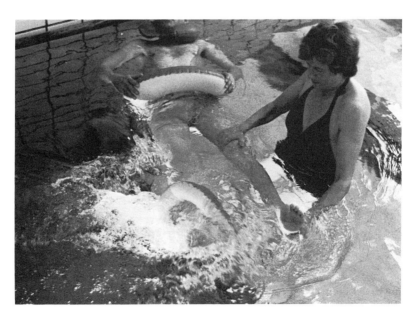

Stabilisations—co-contraction of quadriceps and hamstrings

This technique can be used on any muscle group, but it is frequently required at the knee joint when pain and poor muscle power are the chief problems, particularly in the patient with rheumatoid arthritis. The patient lies comfortably supported in the supine position, the knee to be worked slightly flexed and supported in a pain-free position by the physiotherapist, who stands facing the patient at his feet, one hand around the heel or ankle, the other around the knee. The physiotherapist moves the patient forwards, that is, towards the patient's head through the water, telling him not to let the knee bend. She should be able to see the quadriceps activity and feel the resistance to flexion. The movement through the water is reversed and the patient instructed not to let the knee straighten, again activity in the working muscles—the hamstrings—can be felt, as can the resistance to extension. As the patient learns to respond to the reversal of muscle activity, the speed at which this occurs can be increased by decreased movement of the body in each direction until movement is only minimal and both groups can be felt to be working simultaneously. This procedure can be repeated with the knee in different positions in the pain-free range. Using the isometric work, strengthening and stability of the knee can be improved without painful movement through range.

Combination of isometric (stabilising) and isotonic work for lower extremities

Isotonic activity of one leg whilst the other leg is working isometrically will facilitate the stabilising work. Conversely, if the muscle groups working isometrically are at full strength, this can be used to irradiate into the weaker muscle groups of the other leg working isotonically. Combinations of various patterns can be used, depending upon which muscle groups are weakest and which strongest. The basic technique using one isotonic and one isometric pattern is described.

Right leg flexion, adduction, lateral rotation: isotonic, left leg extension, abduction, medial rotation: isometric (Fig. 6.24)

With the patient lying supported in the supine-lying position, the physiotherapist stands at the patient's feet. Very little movement of the body through the water will occur and the physiotherapist can, therefore, take any position with her feet which will afford maximum stability. She places her right hand on the plantar surface of the patient's left foot which is taken down in the water so that the hip is in a position of extension, abduction and medial rotation. The physiotherapist's left hand is placed on the dorsum of the patient's right foot. The patient is first instructed to push down and outwards with the left leg and to hold it in that position against the resistance of the physiotherapist. Whilst the isometric activity of the left leg is maintained, the patient is asked to flex, adduct and laterally rotate the right leg flexing the knee, dorsi-flexing and inverting the foot. At the end of range, the leg is relaxed, returns to the starting position and the movement is then repeated. The stabilising leg can work isometrically in either a flexion or extension synergy.

As the physiotherapist has only one hand on each leg and both manual contacts are distal, it is not advisable to use isotonic/isometric work as described when pain is a factor. However, the technique is extremely useful when there is weakness in one or two groups, as repeated contractions to the muscles working isotonically can be used with ease and to advantage. Trunk muscles work isometrically and can thus be used also to irradiate into the weaker lower extremity.

Fig. 6.24 Right leg hip flexion, adduction, medial rotation, knee flexion and dorsi flexion: isotonic left leg extension, abduction, medial rotation, knee extension and plantar flexion: isometric

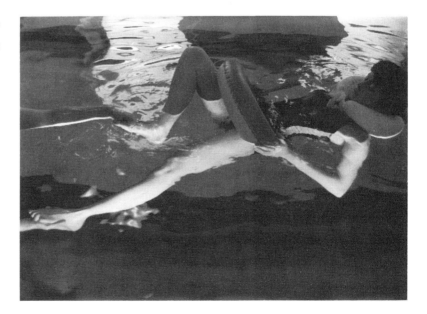

Trunk patterns

Trunk side flexion (Fig. 6.25)

In supine the patient is supported by a body ring and neck collar. One small ring is placed around both ankles so that the legs remain close together. As all trunk patterns involve large movements and (unless the patient is very weak) much muscle activity, it is essential that the physiotherapist stabilises herself well and uses what mechanical advantage she is able to.

Extra stability can be utilised if the physiotherapist stands with her back against the pool wall, which will enable her to brace herself as the patient is moving and she is providing the fixation.

The patient places both hands behind his neck, fingers interlocked, and the physiotherapist standing behind the patient's head positions her hands on his elbows. The top of the patient's head should be as close to the physiotherapist as possible, and she should be as low in the water as possible with her shoulders submerged and her upper arms close into her sides. The patient is asked to take both legs to the right, as he does so the physiotherapist gives pressure to the humeral aspect of the patient's right elbow and to the radio-ulnar aspect on the left as far as possible; the physiotherapist then changes her manual contacts so that she applies pressure to the humeral aspect of the elbow on the left and to the radio-ulnar aspect on the right as the patient takes the legs to the left.

It is most important that, during movement of the trunk, the physiotherapist does not allow any swing of the patient's upper trunk, and that she keeps the top of the patient's head close to her and her upper arms into her sides.

Trunk extension (Fig. 6.26)

The same starting position and manual contacts are used as for trunk side flexion. The patient is asked to turn the right hip uppermost and to pull his legs to the right. He then turns the left hip uppermost and pulls to the left.

Fig. 6.25 Trunk side flexion to the right, fixation at elbows

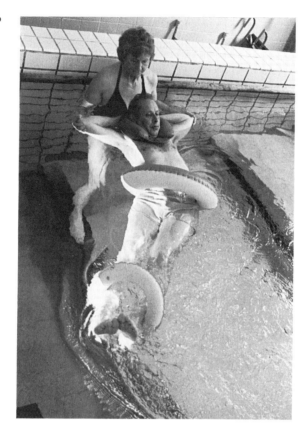

Fig. 6.26 Trunk extension to left, fixation at elbows

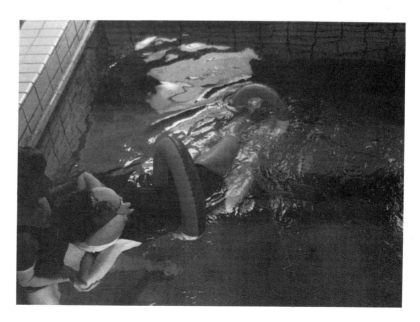

Trunk flexion (Fig. 6.27).

This pattern also commences from the same starting position of patient and physiotherapist. The patient is asked to turn the left hip uppermost and pull the legs to the right. He then turns the right hip uppermost and pulls the legs to the left.

The manual contacts for the above three movements can be varied. Most commonly, the holds need to be more proximal if the patient is weaker, cannot place the hands behind the neck or the physiotherapist wishes to localise the movement. The physiotherapist places her hands on the posterior aspect of the thorax, spreading her hands around the rib cage, below the scapulae, her forearms posterior to the gleno-humeral joints. The pressure and counter-pressure which was used at the elbows is applied in the same way to the thorax and posterior upper trunk (Fig. 6.28).

Alternatively, in order to give more work to the muscles around the shoulder girdle, the arms can be stretched sideways, the physiotherapist holding the patient's upper arms to provide the pressure and counter-pressure. In practice, this is only used in the treatment of children, since with an adult the physiotherapist is positioned at a mechanical disadvantage and fixation is very difficult to provide effectively.

Fig. 6.27 Trunk flexion to right, fixation at elbows

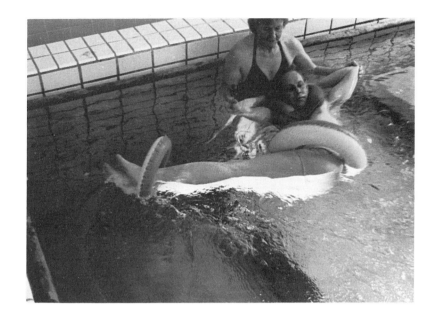

Fig. 6.28 Trunk side flexion to left showing proximal hand hold around scapula area

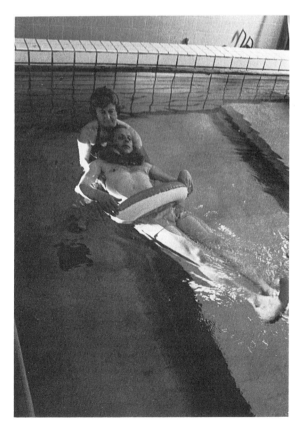

Trunk flexion and extension with rotation in supine

This involves muscle activity not only in the neck and trunk, but also in the full range of movement of the lower extremities. The patient lies supine, supported by a neck collar and body ring. As this is a large movement pattern, the physiotherapist must stabilise herself as well as possible. It is usually advantageous if she stands with her back against the pool wall; she provides fixation for the patient at his feet. Trunk flexion and extension done from this position are best used as a reversal, that is no relaxation occurring at the end of range, the muscle work being changed immediately to the antagonistic pattern.

The physiotherapist places a hand on the dorsum of each foot and tells the patient to pull the feet up, bend the legs, turning the knees to the right, and lift the head to look at the feet. When full flexion is achieved, the physiotherapist lowers the patient's feet in the water and moves her hand holds to the plantar aspect of the feet. The patient is told to turn the knees to the left, put the head back and push, i.e. extend. At the end of the extension range, flexion is again repeated. After a pause the rotation is changed and the patient asked to turn the knees to the left on flexion and to the right on extension (Figs 6.29 and 6.30).

Fig. 6.29 Trunk flexion in supine, total body flexion

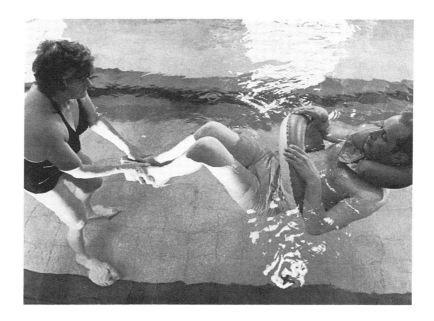

Fig. 6.30 Trunk extension in supine. Note that the physiotherapist has lowered the model's feet in the water and the model is leading the movement with neck extension

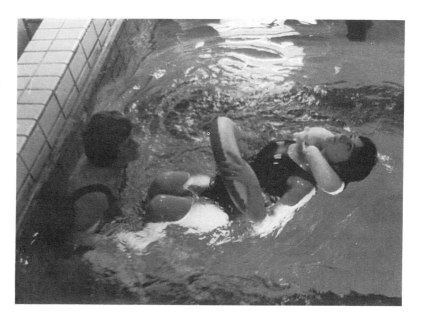

Trunk side flexion in supine with lower extremity fixation
(Fig. 6.31)

With the patient in supine, supported by a neck and body ring (the latter frequently not required), the physiotherapist positions herself between the patient's legs with a hand around each knee (the manual contact can be more proximal or distal depending on need). The patient is asked to take the right hand down the outside of the right leg as far as he can. As he does so, the physiotherapist remains stable, but moves the patient's trunk in an arc through the water to the patient's right. This movement can be fast or slow, depending on the amount of resistance to be offered to the muscle work. When the extreme of movement has been reached, the patient is asked to side flex to the left and take the left hand down the outside of his left leg as the physiotherapist moves him through an arc towards his left. If maximal movement and resistance is required, the physiotherapist, although keeping her feet in position, rotates as far as possible on her own long axis. Extra resistance can be provided by the patient holding his arms in abduction.

Trunk flexion and extension in side-lying (Figs 6.32 and 6.33)

A neck ring is not usually necessary for this exercise as the body ring provides sufficient support. The patient, if lying on the left side, takes the left arm out of the ring and holds the ring with both hands. The physiotherapist positions herself either at the front of the patient or behind him. The former position is the one of choice as it is easier for the patient to hear the commands and the physiotherapist can more easily see the patient's facial expression. With the patient in left side-lying and the physiotherapist in front

Fig. 6.31 Trunk side flexion to the right with fixation at the lower extremities

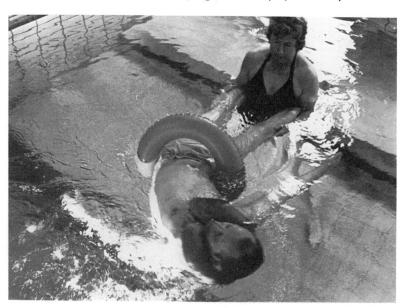

of the patient, she places her right hand under the patient's pelvis and her left hand on the upper aspect (right) of the pelvis. The patient is asked to bend forwards, and as he does so the physiotherapist moves him forwards in an arc through the water, maintaining her stance, but turning on her own long axis. At the extreme of movement the physiotherapist moves her left hand and forearm through 90 degrees so that it lies across the posterior aspect of both thighs. The patient is now asked to extend, leading with the head and right shoulder. The physiotherapist now moves him backwards in an arc through the water.

Fig. 6.32 Trunk flexion in left side-lying. Fixation by physiotherapist at pelvis and thighs

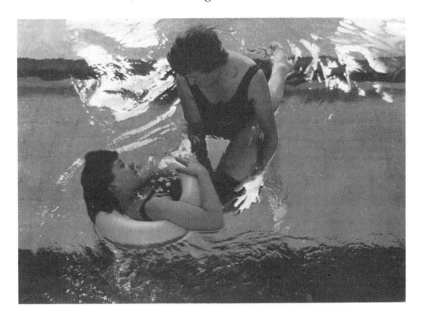

Fig. 6.33 Trunk extension in left side-lying. Fixation at pelvis and thighs. Note physiotherapist's left hand positioned on thighs posteriorly.

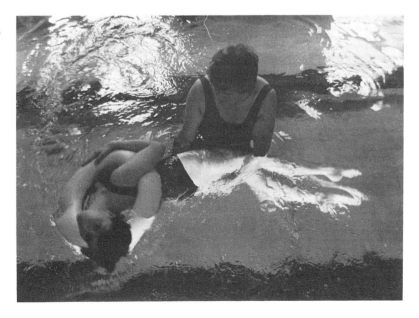

Trunk stabilisation in supine (Fig. 6.34)

The patient lies supine supported by a neck and body ring. The physiotherapist stands between the patient's legs with a hand under each thigh.

It is explained to the patient that he must lie absolutely still and keep his body in a straight line as he is moved through the water. The physiotherapist, maintaining her stance, moves the patient through the water in an arc in one direction, ensuring that the patient maintains the trunk in mid-position and that the movement of the water (bow wave and turbulence) does not cause him to side flex. The direction of the movement through the water is changed, and the patient must again retain the mid-position of the trunk. The speed at which the patient is moved through the water and the distance moved in each direction will depend upon the strength of the trunk muscles and their ability to sustain isometric contraction.

Trunk stabilisation in flexion

The patient commences in supine with a body ring for support. The physiotherapist stands at the patient's feet, holding them firmly together. The patient is asked to lift his head and come halfway to the sitting position in the water. He is then told to hold that position. The physiotherapist now moves the patient in all directions through the water, also moving the legs in relation to the trunk so that a demand is put upon the rotation element in the trunk and lower extremity muscle groups.

Fig. 6.34 Trunk stabilisation in supine. Model retains the 'mid'-position as he is moved through the water to the left.

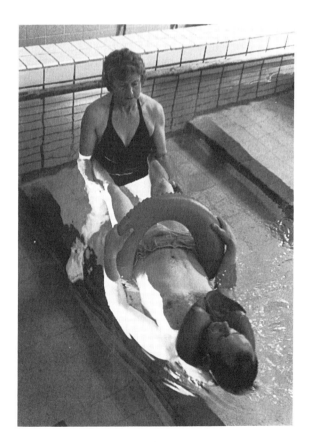

Upper extremity patterns

Right arm abduction and lateral rotation (Fig. 6.35)

Working from the starting position, as described, with this particular pattern it is not possible to include a flexion/extension component, the movement commencing from the neutral position.

The patient lies supine with neck and body supporting rings and with a small ring around both ankles. The physiotherapist stands on the right of the patient at the level of his shoulder; he lies with his arms at his sides. The physiotherapist places her right hand on the dorsum of the patient's right hand. The physiotherapist's right hand can be used to provide more fixation and can be placed on the outer aspect of the patient's arm. More usually, the physiotherapist will use her left arm to prevent excessive movement at the shoulder joint and so enable the movement to occur through the pain-free range. She, therefore, places her left arm under the patient's scapular region, with her hand resting on the left side of the shoulder girdle.

The patient is asked to push his trunk away from his arm dorsiflexing his wrist and fingers and laterally rotating at the glenohumeral joint. The physiotherapist provides maximum fixation with her left hand; she leans forwards and the patient moves through part of a circle. At the end of the required range, the patient relaxes, the physiotherapist walks forward so returning the patient's arm to his side. The movement is then repeated.

Right arm adduction and medial rotation (Fig. 6.36)

This pattern is the reverse of the above; the patient lies with his right arm abducted as far as is comfortable for him, the elbow, wrist and fingers extended. The physiotherapist places her right hand in the palm of the patient, asking him to grip her hand, turn the arm inwards and pull his body towards his arm. The physiotherapist leans backwards and again the patient moves through the arc of a circle.

Fig. 6.35 End of range, right shoulder abduction and lateral rotation

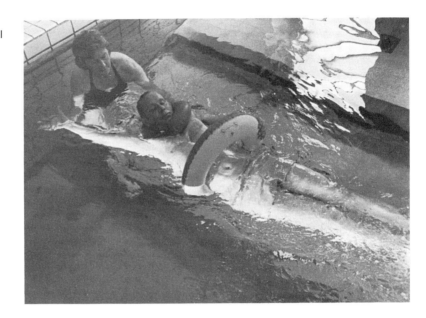

Fig. 6.36 Right shoulder, adduction and medial rotation, mid-range

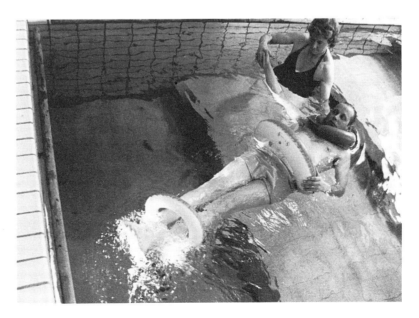

Left arm extension, abduction and medial rotation (Fig. 6.37)

The patient lies in the prone position supported by a body ring and small ring around both ankles. A neck collar worn the opposite way round can be used, but is not usually necessary and also tends to interfere with the movement at the shoulder. The physiotherapist stands at the patient's head, facing him; the patient's left shoulder is flexed (i.e. in elevation) and the physiotherapist places her left hand in the patient's left hand. The patient is asked to keep the elbow straight, grip the physiotherapist's hand and pull his arm downwards and outwards. As he does so, he moves forwards through the water, his left shoulder passing the left shoulder of the physiotherapist as end of range is reached. As the elbow is kept straight throughout the movement, the physiotherapist must ensure that she moves her left hand (holding the patient's left hand) downwards in the water as he moves through middle range. The physiotherapist uses her right hand to guide the patient through the water if this is necessary.

Left arm flexion adduction and lateral rotation

The starting position is as above, the patient has his left arm at his side. The physiotherapist places her left hand on the dorsum of the patient's left wrist, her left shoulder is beside his left shoulder. The patient is asked to push away, keeping the elbow straight. He thus moves backwards through the water until the shoulder is flexed in elevation. The physiotherapist uses her right hand to assist the movement of the body through the water, particularly guiding the adduction component.

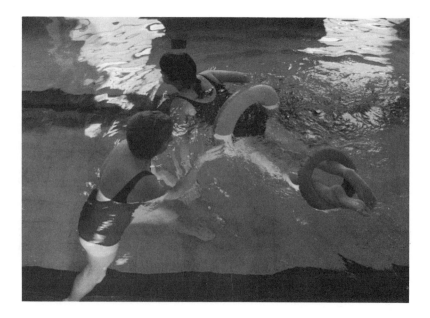

Fig. 6.37 Left shoulder, extension, abduction and medial rotation

Left arm extension, adduction and medial rotation (Fig. 6.38)

The prone position is again used for this pattern, the physiotherapist stands at the patient's head, facing him. The patient's left arm is flexed at the shoulder and in slight abduction. The physiotherapist places her left hand in the patient's left hand. The patient is asked to grip the physiotherapist's hand, keep the elbow straight and pull the arm down through the water to his right hip. He thus moves through the water, his right shoulder passing the physiotherapist's right shoulder as he moves to the end of range.

Left arm flexion, abduction and lateral rotation

The starting position is that which is reached at the end of range of the preceding pattern. The physiotherapist slips her hand onto the dorsum of the patient's left hand. The patient is asked to push away from the physiotherapist, and travels backwards through the water as he moves through range to full elevation. The elbow is again kept straight throughout the movement and the physiotherapist moves her hand downwards in the water as he passes through the mid-range. The physiotherapist's right hand is again guiding the movement of the patient through the water.

Bilateral symmetrical arm patterns

The preceding four patterns of movement can be used bilaterally with the patient in the prone position. The elbows are kept straight, and to allow for full range to occur the physiotherapist must be slightly to one side or other as the patient reaches inner range in the extension patterns.

Fig. 6.38 Left shoulder, extension, adduction and medial rotation, early in range

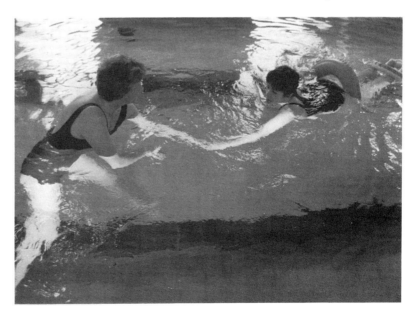

Bilateral flexion and extension of arms—'heaving and thrusting'
(Figs 6.39, 6.40 and 6.41)

The patient is supported in the supine position, the physiotherapist at the patient's head. The patient flexes his elbows and the physiotherapist holds both of his hands in a palmar grip. The patient is asked to push away from the physiotherapist, as he does so extending the elbows and flexing at the gleno-humeral joints. The physiotherapist leans into the movement and steps forwards as the end of range is reached. The patient relaxes, the arms are returned to the starting position and the movement repeated. For the reverse of the pattern, with the arms fully elevated and elbows extended, the patient is asked to flex both elbows and pull towards the physiotherapist, thus extending at the gleno-humeral joints. She must lean backwards as he does so and also must enable the patient's head to move towards one of her shoulders. The physiotherapist must ensure, whilst doing these two patterns, that she keeps low in the water with her fixation, otherwise there will be a tendency for the patient's head and shoulders to be submerged.

Fig. 6.39 Starting position for bilateral flexion of shoulders with elbow extension— 'thrusting'

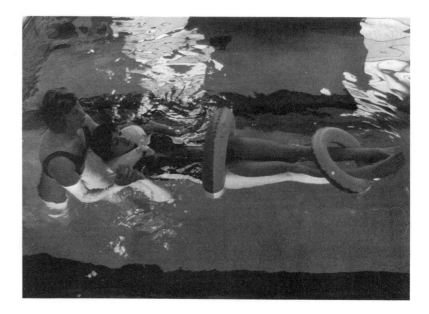

REFERENCES

Bolton E 1971 A technique of resistive exercise adapted for a small pool. Physiotherapy 57:10
Davis B C 1971 A technique of resistive exercise in the treatment pool. Physiotherapy 57:10
Harrison R A 1980 A quantitative approach to muscle strengthening in the hydrotherapy pool. Physiotherapy 66:2
Harrison R A, Allard L L 1982 An attempt to quantify the resistance produced using the Bad Ragaz ring method. Physiotherapy 68:10

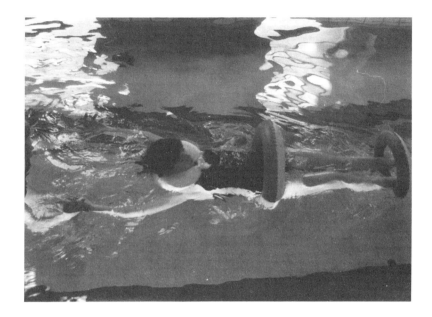

Fig. 6.40 End of range 'thrusting': note extension of wrists and fingers

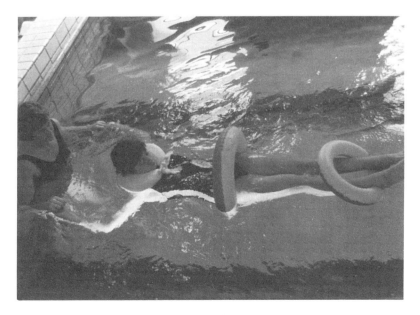

Fig. 6.41 Extension with adduction of shoulders, flexion of elbows, wrists and fingers— 'heaving'

7

Partial weight-bearing and gait re-education

The hydrotherapy pool provides an ideal environment for the re-education of gait. It is particularly appropriate for patients who have been immobilised or on bed rest for any length of time, and also for those with weakness of trunk and lower extremities or poor balance. However, due to the physical properties of water which have been discussed in Chapter 4 and elsewhere, the activity of walking in water differs to some extent to walking on dry land.

PARTIAL WEIGHT-BEARING

In the early re-education of walking the pool provides the physiotherapist with a means of progressing partial weight-bearing by small increments as well as providing a method in which the amount of weight passing through the limb can be assessed. In this respect it is unique, for in the physiotherapy department, unless one has access to sophisticated transducer apparatus, this is not possible. One may demonstrate to the patient by the use of bath-room scales, for example, how much weight he should put through the limb, but once walking begins, this is outside the control of the physiotherapist and dependent only upon the patient's understanding and willingness to comply.

We know from the application of Archimedes' principle (p. 58) that when the human body is partially immersed in the hydrotherapy pool it will experience an upthrust equal to the weight of the water which the immersed part displaces. Since the combined specific gravities of its various component tissues give the body an apparent specific gravity of just less than 1, the upthrust can be thought of as cancelling out the effect of gravity on the immersed parts. To all intents, the weight passing through the lower limbs will be equal to the combined weights of the parts of the body which are still out of the water.

The only figure which has appeared in the literature to give physiotherapists a quantitative idea of the weight which passes through the legs during partial immersion has been that for immersion to the level of the neck, which is usually said to give partial weight-bearing of 10%. Measurements made by Harrison and Bulstrode (1986) have shown that working approximations can be made for different depths of immersion.

Immersion to the levels of C7, xiphisternum and ASIS give percentage weight-bearing of approximately 10%, 30% and 50% respectively.

It must be remembered that the figures given for partial weight-bearing are only approximate and will vary slightly from person to person according to their physical build, but they will provide a useful indication to the practising physiotherapist of forces involved.

It will be obvious that when the subject is standing in the pool with the weight distributed equally between both legs, the effective weight, as described above, will be divided equally between both lower limbs so that a person immersed to the level of the seventh cervical vertebra will have approximately 5% of the body weight passing through each leg. If, however, one leg is lifted from the bottom of the pool then the whole 10% will pass through the supporting limb.

When standing on both feet the stress on the feet, ankles, tibiae, knee joints, femurs and hip joints will be equal to the weight as described, and in one-legged standing the same will also apply, but with the exception of the hip joint. This is because during standing on one leg, the body weight, passing through the mid-line, exerts a turning force on the pelvis, pivoting it on the fixed head of the weight-bearing femur. If the hip abductors of that side are weak or ineffectual then the hip at the other side drops. If, however, as is normal, the abductors of the hip contract strongly so that the pelvis remains level, the hip joint is subjected not only to the body weight passing through it, but also to the pull of the abductors. Were the hip joint half way between the mid-line and the origins of the abductors, then the pull of the abductors would be equal and opposite and the femoral head would be subjected to a force of $2 \times$ the body weight. In fact, the hip abductors are working at a mechanical disadvantage and the distance of the body mid-line to the hip joint is approximately $2.4 \times$ the distance from the abductor origins to the hip joint. The total force to which the hip joint will be subjected when the subject stands on one leg will, therefore, be of the order of $3 \times$ the body weight (Strange 1965).

The same principle will apply when standing on one leg and partially immersed in water, when the force through the hip joint will be about $3 \times$ the weight of the part of the body above the water.

The observations above relate to the static position, and it must be remembered that the forces through the limb will increase when walking commences. This force will become greater as speed of walking increases.

Discrepancy in leg length

Some of the conditions which the physiotherapist will wish to treat in the pool by partial weight-bearing will have a true shortening of one leg as part of the clinical picture. Examples would be osteoarthrosis of the hip joint, arthrodesis of the knee and some fractures.

On dry land the patient will probably wear adapted footwear to compensate for the shortening:and it is necessary to provide an equivalent for use in the hydrotherapy pool. Unless provision is made for this, equal weight-bearing through both legs is not possible and abnormalities of gait cannot be corrected and re-educated.

The need for such a raise will be seen when the patient is assessed, probably at a pre-pool attendance, and this will give time for a heel cup or sandal to be made before the patient attends for his first treatment.

Raises of various patterns have been devised by physiotherapists for their patients (see Fig. 7.1), and these need not be elaborate to be effective. They can be made of wood or Plastazote, but it must be remembered that if made of a buoyant material, the heel cup will need to be weighted or it will act as a float and, rather than improve the gait, will interfere with the walking pattern.

Unless the raise fits very well and is particularly securely fixed to the patient's foot, it is safer to remove it before the patient leaves the pool.

Fig. 7.1 Heel raise made of wood and thermoplastic splinting material with webbing strap and velcro fastening

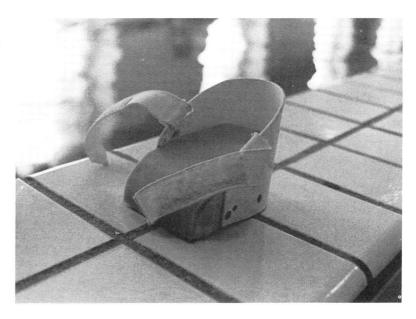

NORMAL GAIT

As walking consists of the translation of the centre of gravity horizontally, muscle action must exert both a horizontal force to move the centre of gravity and a vertical force to prevent it from falling due to the effect of gravity. Walking in water makes one of these easier and the other more difficult. Because water has a greater density than air, the effect of gravity is reduced and the muscle activity required to support the body weight is less. On the other hand, the density of water compared with air increases the resistance to the movement of the body and extremities, making greater demands on the muscles performing that movement.

Following immobilisation or for patients with pain and consequent muscle weakness, the advantage of walking in water can be summarised as follows:

Joints which are painful whilst walking on dry land are less painful when the patient walks in water because of the effective reduction in body weight due to the support provided by the water. There is less demand on the muscles to support the body weight, but at the same time the water provides increased resistance to the other muscle actions of walking.

Before studying the effect of the activity on joints and muscles which occurs during walking in water, it is relevant to discuss the major events occurring in normal gait on dry land.

Gait can be defined as the translation of the centre of gravity of the human body through space along a pathway requiring the least expenditure of energy.

The gait cycle is that sequence of events which occur from heel strike of one foot through to the next heel strike of that same foot. There are two phases: stance and swing (Fig. 7.2).

The stance phase occurs for approximately 60% of the cycle, the swing phase for the remaining 40%. A period of double support, when both feet are in contact with the ground, lasts for approximately 15% of the cycle, although this will vary considerably with the speed of walking. The period of double support decreases the faster the subject walks, until there is no period of double support, at which point the subject is running.

The reader is referred to other texts for the detailed analysis of joint and muscle activity, but a brief summary is described.

Stance phase

Stance is predominantly an extension activity and commences with heel strike. At this point the hip is slightly flexed, knee extended, foot dorsiflexed and toes extended. As the trunk moves forwards over the supporting leg to mid-stance, the hip extends, the knee flexes to a maximum of 15 degrees at mid-stance, and the foot and toes plantar flex, although this is minimal in the phase from heel strike to mid-stance.

From mid-stance to toe-off the centre of gravity of the body moves in front of the supporting leg. The hip extends further, the

Fig. 7.2 The phases of the normal gait pattern

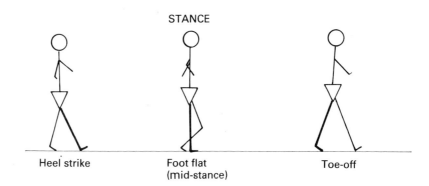

STANCE

Heel strike   Foot flat (mid-stance)   Toe-off

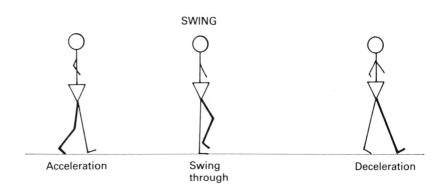

SWING

Acceleration   Swing through   Deceleration

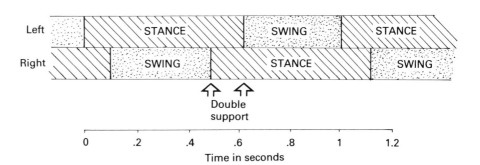

knee remains in approximately 5 °–15 ° of flexion, and the foot and toes move further into plantar flexion.

Swing phase

Flexion predominates throughout swing from toe-off through acceleration and deceleration, although the muscle activity is primarily in the extensor groups where both concentric and eccentric work occurs.

After toe-off has occurred, the hip and knee flex, and the foot and toes dorsiflex during the acceleration phase. As the leg passes the mid-position and deceleration occurs the hip extensors work eccentrically, the knee extends, the foot and toes remaining dorsiflexed.

In the early stage of stance the dorsiflexors, quadriceps, hamstrings, hip abductors and adductors, gluteus maximus and the trunk extensors are contracting strongly. By 30% of the cycle, most of this activity has dropped off and the only major group working strongly by mid-stance are the calf muscles, although the hip abductors continue working to approximately 40% of the cycle. In the last 10% of stance the dorsiflexors, quadriceps, hamstrings, hip adductors, gluteus maximus and trunk extensors are again actively working and continue into the first 10 to 20% of swing. At toe-off, that is at the end of stance, the hip flexors work strongly to help initiate swing. By the time mid-swing has been reached, activity is mainly discernible in the dorsiflexors, hip flexors and trunk extensors, activity having dropped off in the other groups. By the last 10% of swing all previously mentioned muscle groups except the calf muscles become active again and continue through the final stage of swing into stance.

Apart from the movement and muscle activity in the lower extremities, the movement of the pelvis is of considerable significance in the normal gait pattern. Indeed, three of the basic determinants of the gait pattern of the normal subject are related to adjustments that are made at the pelvis in relation to lower extremity and trunk activity (Saunders et al 1953).

1. Pelvic rotation

As the pelvis rotates forwards the movement occurs at each hip joint which moves (on swing) from relative medial rotation to relative lateral rotation in stance. There is reciprocal rotation of the shoulders and, therefore, also arm swing to compensate. Pelvic rotation allows for lengthening of the stride without an excessive drop of the centre of gravity.

2. Pelvic tilt

The pelvis tilts down from the weight-bearing (stance) leg approximately 5 ° at mid-stance. This reduces the rise in centre of gravity.

3. Lateral movement of the pelvis

There is a shift of the body weight from the pelvis to the stance leg, that is a horizontal movement of the centre of gravity of approximately 5 cm at mid-stance.

GAIT IN THE MEDIUM OF WATER

When the subject walks in water, the pattern and events of the gait cycle, together with the joint action and pelvic motion, are identical to those occurring when the subject walks on dry land as described above. However, muscle activity is clearly different due to the effect of buoyancy.

Extensive analytical studies of gait have been done over the years, and with the use of computerised infra-red photographs, cinematography, pedo-barometry and various other electronic equipment, many more parameters of human gait are being studied. As far as the authors can discover, however, no study has yet been made of the muscle activity occurring when a human subject walks in water. The description that follows, therefore, is based on observation, experience and an applied knowledge of hydrodynamics.

The activity described is with the subject walking in water of a depth where the water surface comes to the level of the nipple line.

Stance phase

Throughout the stance phase, from heel strike to toe-off, buoyancy will exert little effect on the joint and muscle activity in the supporting limb. However, as the trunk (in fact the whole body) is moving through water the effects of the bow wave and turbulence in water will provide resistance to the forward movement. There will thus be a need for the subject to lean forwards in order to push against the resistance of the water. The consequent effect on muscle activity will be an increase in work in the trunk flexors. As the stance limb, particularly the foot, is the fixed or more stable part over which the body is moving, there will be an increased activity in the muscle groups of the lower extremity, particularly the extensors. It is the extensor groups which will have a propulsive effect and thus assist in moving the body against the weight of the water.

Swing phase

At toe-off, which initiates the swing phase, buoyancy assists flexion of the leg. However, the acceleration phase of swing is slowed considerably as the effect of the movement of the limb through the water is to produce turbulence and the limb has to be carried through against the resistance of the water. It is reasonable to suppose, therefore, that there is an increased demand on the hip flexors and rectus femoris to bring the limb through mid-swing. The dorsiflexors also work against the increased resistance of the water through swing. Once the limb is past mid-swing, the effects of buoyancy shift. The hip flexors are now assisted by the upthrust, and knee extension which commences just after mid-swing is also assisted. At the end of deceleration, when the hip is flexed and the knee extended, buoyancy resists hip extension as the limb moves downwards to heel strike.

It will be appreciated from the above description of gait on dry land and in the water, that walking re-education in water can be used to advantage, particularly during the early stages of rehabilitation. The muscle and joint activity occurring can be made easier or more difficult depending on need, by utilising in particular the effects of turbulence, the resistance of water and buoyancy.

STANDING ACTIVITIES

There are many activities in the standing position in which the properties of water can be used to advantage at different stages of the patient's rehabilitation. The depth of water in which these activities are performed will depend upon whether there is a need to relieve weight through the extremities and upon the extent to which buoyancy is to be used to assist or resist the movement. In shallower water, buoyancy will have less effect. It is preferable for the patient to work on these activities in the deeper part of the pool with the water level approximately at the nipple line. Simple apparatus may be used, such as rings and Plastazote floats. If one or both lower extremities are weak, it may be found helpful to use weighted sandals as these help the patient to keep the feet on the floor of the pool when standing.

Hip extension

The patient stands facing the hand rail which he holds with both hands. The physiotherapist stabilises the pelvis and the patient is requested to extend the leg backwards, lifting it as high as possible. A ring containing a small amount of air can be fixed in a figure of eight fashion around the patient's foot and ankle to assist the movement and to increase the stretching effect to the structures anterior to the hip joint.

Hip flexion (Fig. 7.3)

Very occasionally it may be necessary to increase the patient's ability to flex at the hip. This may be because of weakness of the flexors due to a neurological condition or, for instance, following total replacement of the hip. Lack of hip flexion can, in particular, cause difficulties climbing stairs. In water, particularly when weakness and lack of range are considerable, hip flexion can be encouraged with ease and no discomfort. The patient stands facing the rail which he holds for stability. A ring containing a small amount of air is positioned on his foot and, with the guidance of the physiotherapist, the hip is flexed as far as possible, with the ring providing assistance. As the movement improves, the ring is discarded and the patient, in the deeper part of the pool, works on the movement by placing the foot up a step or onto a small block. To progress further, this activity is performed in shallower water until finally the patient is able to leave the pool by the steps.

Hip and knee flexion—extension

The patient is positioned for the commencement of this movement as above. The patient is asked to flex the leg forwards at hip and knee as fully as possible and then to extend downwards and backwards. Most frequently this exercise is done using resistance to the extension component and assistance to flexion. The patient places his foot in a ring which has sufficient air in it to provide the required resistance or assistance. The ring can be placed around the foot in a figure of eight or, if this is not possible because of the amount of air or size of ring, the ring is placed on the sole of the patient's foot.

Fig. 7.3 Buoyancy used as assistance to hip flexion

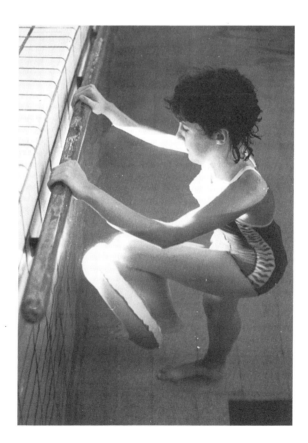

If buoyant apparatus is used to assist flexion or to resist extension, the utmost care must be taken to give a full explanation to the patient. The patient must understand that as the limb is brought into flexion, unless he maintains control over the movement by eccentric work of the hip extensors, a forceful, uncontrolled flexion movement will occur. It is likewise important that the physiotherapist does not use a ring with too much air or too large a float. By varying the amount of buoyancy in the apparatus, the movement can be made stronger. If necessary, the physiotherapist can assist the patient to control the movement by placing her foot over that of the patient's in the ring.

STANDING BALANCE

The patient stands in the water, away from the side of the pool or any hand rail or other piece of fixed apparatus. The depth of the water is significant for this manoeuvre, as the deeper the water the more difficult it will be for the patient to retain his balance. The exercise can thus be progressed by commencing in shallower water and then moving into the deeper part of the pool. The physiotherapist creates an area of turbulence by moving her hands in the water at the level of the patient's lower trunk or pelvis. A pair of paddles (table tennis bats) can be used to create a greater degree of turbulence. Since the patient will have a tendency to be 'pulled' towards the turbulent area, if working for general balance reactions in the upright position it is important that the turbulent effect is created at different aspects of the body in turn. As turbulence creates a drag effect on the body and tends to pull the body

Fig. 7.4 Turbulence used to assist gait re-education

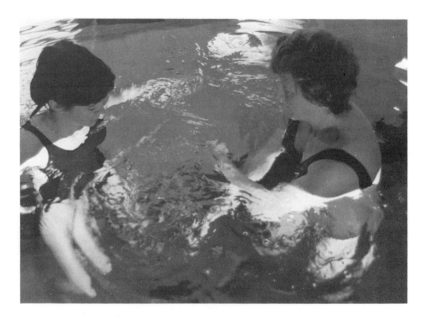

towards the turbulent area, it can be seen that this is a very useful means of encouraging weight transference. If, for example, a patient is reluctant, when walking, to put his body weight over one leg, by using turbulence, weight-bearing can be encouraged on that side together with the lateral movement of the pelvis and trunk.

For the child or adult who, in standing, shows excessive extensor tone causing him to lean backwards, the generation of a turbulent area in front of the trunk above the level of the umbilicus, will encourage a more flexed standing position, and with verbal encouragement the patient should also be able to bring the upper extremities to a more anterior position. In cases of excessive forward leaning, turbulence is created behind the patient.

WALKING ACTIVITIES

Although to a certain extent the muscle work involved in walking in water is different when compared to that of walking on dry land, water has a considerable advantage as a medium for gait training. This is especially true in the early stages of rehabilitation. For the patient who is moderately to severely paralysed, or who has been immobilised for a long period of time, the early commencement of pool therapy with walking re-education is particularly useful. The ability to begin gait re-education in water earlier than would be possible on dry land exposes the patient to a variety of stimuli which are activated by the assumption of the upright position and of bi-pedal locomotion. Both feet are in contact with the floor of the pool and, therefore, exeroceptive and proprioceptive stimuli are being received and extensor muscle groups, in particular, stimulated. Postural reactions and balance mechanisms are stimulated, whether or not the patient holds the hand rail. It may occasionally be necessary to support the knees by the use of polythene back splints, and to use Plastazote sandals with or without weights. These additional supports help the patient to retain the upright posture and do not decrease the stimuli nor the response mechanisms. In spite of some altered muscle work, particularly in the swing phase in walking, early walking in water enables the patient to regain the 'picture' or dynamic image of this functional activity. Normal pathways are stimulated in relation to the activity occurring in joints and in the muscles which have both static and kinetic functions.

The use of hand rails

As on dry land, the patient often requires extra stability, or it may be that the physiotherapist wishes to reinforce muscle activity and so needs the patient to use his upper extremities to act as a means of fixation, stabilisation and reinforcement. All hydrotherapy pools should have a hand rail which passes round the pool at water level. Many pools have an area designated for gait re-education, where a second rail at the same level will be positioned allowing an appropriate space between. Of necessity, the rails are placed at a height which is not as functional as parallel bars on dry land. However, they are nonetheless useful, and serve their purpose satisfactorily. Progression of gait activities in water usually commences with the use of two rails, then one, and subsequently with the patient free of any support.

Manual resistance (Fig. 7.5)

Resistance can be given manually by the physiotherapist in much the same way as on dry land. Most commonly, resistance and guidance are given at the pelvis or at the shoulder girdle. In water, another useful point of load is the patient's foot, the physiotherapist using her own foot to provide the resistance. This is quite comfortable for the patient, and easy and accurate for the physiotherapist.

Fig. 7.5 Manual resistance applied to pelvis during gait re-education

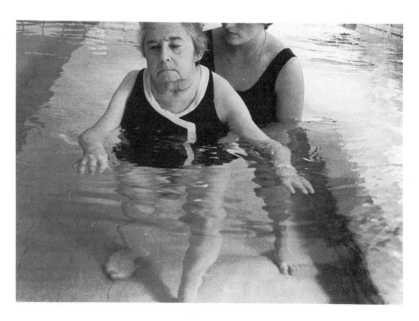

Other means of altering resistance

Changing direction

If, on walking forwards, the patient is asked to change direction and walk backwards, as well as the change in muscle work of the trunk and lower extremities, the water around the body becomes more turbulent due to reversal of the movement. Thus, at the time of reversal, retention of balance is more difficult, and becomes more so, the sharper the reversal of movement.

Speed

The faster the patient walks the more turbulence is generated; he must thus lean in the direction in which he is moving to push against the resistance of the water.

Equipment

A paddle (table tennis bat) held in each hand with the broad surface facing forwards—backwards and the elbows held straight will greatly add to the resistance offered in walking, due to the less streamlined body shape which is presented to the water. The size of the paddles can be altered and so have a further influence on the resistance provided.

GAIT EXERCISES

Walking activities in the pool can be divided into major categories:
1. Those which emphasise the precise elements of the gait cycle which are causing the deficiencies in the patient's gait on dry land.
2. Those which are used for further re-education of lower limb and trunk muscle groups in the upright posture.
   Both these types of activity are for the purpose of improving gait, but the first group is more specific to the pattern of gait.

1. Elements of gait cycle

Initiation of swing phase

The toe-off component of the swing phase can be readily worked in the pool. Due to buoyancy the body weight is in effect reduced so that weak or inefficient plantar flexors, in particular, can function more easily. Holding onto one or two rails, the patient is told to emphasise the lift onto the toes and push off at each step.

Assistance can be given manually by the physiotherapist at the pelvis if necessary.

Weight transference to stance leg

To encourage correct transference of weight from the pelvis onto the affected side (side to which patient does not correctly transfer his weight), the physiotherapist creates an area of turbulence on that side, progressing forwards with the patient.

Stride length

As the body weight is effectively reduced when standing in water and flexion of the leg is assisted in part of the swing phase, it is normally much easier for the patient to walk with equal stride length. The patient can work on this by himself, if necessary, and monitor his own performance by stepping across an equal number of floor tiles with each step.

Reciprocal rotation of shoulder girdle and trunk

Two hand rails must be used. The patient is instructed to extend the left arm and grip the rail as far forward as he can without leaning his trunk forward. He then takes as large a step as possible with the right leg without moving the right arm or left leg. This is followed by the transference of weight onto the right leg, the right arm is extended and then the left leg, progressing along the bars.

2. Re-education of trunk and lower extremity muscle groups

Strengthening of hip abductors

The patient stands facing the hand rail, holding it with two hands. The physiotherapist stands at the side of the patient and places her foot on the lateral aspect of the patient's right foot. The physiotherapist can place her hand on the side of the patient's pelvis or chest wall for added resistance at the foot. The patient is asked to take a large step to the right against resistance and then to bring the left leg to the right. It is important that the physiotherapist, as well as giving resistance to the movement, ensures that the body weight is brought over the right leg as the left leg is adducted. Verbal reinforcement is frequently necessary.

Strengthening of hip adductors

This is similar to the above, the physiotherapist placing her foot on the inner aspect of the patient's heel. She stabilises the patient by placing a hand on the pelvis on the opposite side.

Strengthening of hip and trunk extensors

The patient stands holding the two hand rails, although one is frequently sufficient. The physiotherapist is behind the patient and places her foot on the patient's heel. He is then asked to take a large step backwards with the right leg. The same is repeated on the left leg. To obtain more work from the trunk extensors, the physiotherapist gives added manual resistance at the shoulder girdle.

'Plaiting'

This activity involves alternate abduction and adduction, manual resistance being given at the pelvis if required. The patient, facing the hand rail and holding it with both hands, steps to the side with the left leg, and places it lateral to the right leg. The patient again steps sideways with the left leg, and adducts the right leg, this time in front of the left leg and so continues.

As the subject walks in progressively deeper water he increasingly uses his arms to assist in propelling himself forwards. If he is instructed to place his arms behind his back, he compensates for lack of use of these extremities by increasing the movement of the upper trunk. This phenomenon can be used to advantage when endeavouring to gain more trunk mobility and to strengthen the trunk rotators.

REFERENCES

Harris R, McInnes M 1963 Exercises in water. In Licht S (ed) Medical hydrology. E. Licht, New Haven, Connecticut, p 207–217
Harrison R A, Bulstrode S 1987 Percentage weight bearing during partial immersion in the hydrotherapy pool. Physiotherapy Practice 3: 60–63
Murdoch G (ed) 1970 Prosthetic and orthotic practice. Edward Arnold, London
Saunders J B de C M, Inman V T, Eberhart H D 1953 The major determinant in normal and pathological gait. Journal of Bone and Joint Surgery 35-A: 543–553
Strange F G St C 1965 The hip. William Heinemann, London, p 26

8

Treatment of specific conditions

Pool therapy can be used to great advantage in the rehabilitation programmes of patients with a variety of conditions, both neurological and non-neurological. For some patients with chronic disease such as rheumatoid arthritis and ankylosing spondylitis, regular periods of daily, or three times a week, pool therapy of between three and six weeks can help considerably in maintaining joint range and muscle strength. It is much more desirable to treat such patients periodically, than to keep them on pool therapy for several months once or twice a week.

Pool therapy should always be used in conjunction with dry land physiotherapy. It is most frequently used in the early stages of a patient's treatment programme, particularly following fractures and surgery as soon as a period of immobilisation is completed, or after the acute stage of a disease. This is because of the considerable advantages of warmth and buoyancy, making it easier for the physiotherapist to handle the patient and providing a comfortable medium for the patient in which he is able to move with greater ease than on dry land and where the warmth of the water reduces any pain which might be present.

As the patient's treatment progresses and muscle strength and joint mobility are improved, pool therapy sessions should be decreased and dry land activities increased, both in intensity and diversity. More time should be spent on functional activities, specific activities of daily living and the patient's work tolerance built up. As the programme progresses, pool therapy will cease to contribute any specific advantage and the patient will spend all his time in the physiotherapy and occupational therapy departments. Swimming can often continue to be of general therapeutic value, but should not require the time of a physiotherapist since the patient can either attend the local swimming baths or, if the hospital pool is large enough, can swim there providing there are responsible able-bodied staff in the area.

In this chapter the use of pool therapy for patients with specific conditions is described. The pathology is described only briefly.

The reader is referred to other texts for the detailed pathology of the conditions. Signs and symptoms are described and the use of pool therapy related to them.

It is important for all physiotherapists to realise that pool therapy is simply a further treatment modality available for their use in the same way as ice, exercise, ultrasound, mobilisation and manipulation, etc. It is, therefore, accepted that it is the physiotherapist who must decide when and for how long and how often the patient should be treated in the pool, and if, indeed, pool therapy will be of any value for that particular patient. It is important, however, that if the physiotherapist is in any doubt or is unclear from reading the patient's medical notes about the patient's general condition, she should discuss this with the doctor responsible. This is particularly important in relation to the condition of the patient's cardiovascular system. It may be that the patient has an open wound, and although a water occlusive dressing and plaster can be applied, even this may not be considered sufficient protection for the patient or provide sufficient protection for other patients if the wound is infected. In these circumstances, the physiotherapist should always discuss these problems with the referring doctor concerned and if necessary the microbiologist.

OSTEOARTHROSIS

Patients with osteoarthrosis of weight-bearing joints who require treatment by physiotherapy and hydrotherapy are less in number than they were formerly because of the success of joint replacement surgery and the consequent decline in conservative treatment. Even so, there will always be some patients for whom surgery is contra-indicated as well as those who require treatment whilst waiting their turn for surgery.

Hydrotherapy forms a useful part of the treatment of both these groups of patients, particularly for muscle strengthening and, also, for those who will not be having surgery, for the mobilisation of stiff joints.

The aims of treatment are:
1. Relief of pain
2. Increase of range of movement
3. Strengthening of weak muscle groups
4. Re-education of function—walking, stairs, standing, sitting.

Relief of pain

Direct relief of pain brought about by the warmth of the water on the sensory cutaneous nerve endings is temporary and the pain will probably soon return after the treatment ends, as will pain lost due to relaxation of muscle spasm.

The usefulness of this aspect of the treatment should not be underestimated, however, for the patient is able to do the mobilising and strengthening exercises more effectively and to work harder whilst the pain is decreased during pool treatment.

Increasing range of movement

Limitation of movement in this condition as in other arthritic conditions may be due to any or all of the following:
1. Pain
2. Muscle spasm
3. Contraction of periarticular fibrous tissue
4. Bony changes

Relief of pain and muscle spasm

These two are physiologically linked and, as stated above, the relief of pain will tend to decrease protective spasm which in turn further reduces pain. In addition to the warmth of the water, gentle rhythmical movements within the pain-free range carried out in a buoyancy supporting position will help to relax such 'tight' muscles.

Example. To induce relaxation of the hip adductors the patient is placed in a supine float-support lying position and slow rhythmical ab- and adduction movements of the hip are encouraged. The movement should begin well within the pain-free range and gradually be increased, taking care that no sharp pain is provoked.

In this position the patient can be encouraged to assess his progress by watching his feet in relation to the tiles on the side of the pool when he will be able to see for himself whether he is increasing his range of movement.

In addition to this type of exercise it may be appropriate for some patients if hold relax techniques are introduced. For the hip joint the Bad Ragaz ab- and adduction patterns are particularly suitable (see p. 101).

Stretching of soft tissue contractures

The physiotherapist is attempting here to stretch fibrous tissue which is limiting joint movement, and obviously this cannot be attempted until any muscle spasm which is present has been released. If spasm is still present then the muscle will limit the movement before the fibrous tissue is put on stretch. This stage will always, therefore, be preceded by exercises aimed at relaxing muscle as described above.

The stretching may be applied as a continuous sustained force, and a technique for using floats as a passive stretching agent is described in the treatment of ankylosing spondylitis (p. 145).

A different approach to controlled sustained stretching by floats is illustrated in the following example.

Example. The aim of this exercise is to apply a stretching force to the front of the hip joint where there is a small degree of hip flexion deformity.

The patient stands holding the rail of the pool as illustrated in Figure 8.1, with his feet about 0.5 m away from the wall of the pool. He is then told to bring his hips forward to try to touch the wall, at the same time keeping his knees straight and not moving his feet to assume the position shown in Figure 8.2. This movement is not, of course, limited to the hip joint, since there will also be extension of the lumbar spine. In practice, however, it does stretch

Fig. 8.1 Hip stretching, position 1   **Fig. 8.2** Hip stretching, position 2

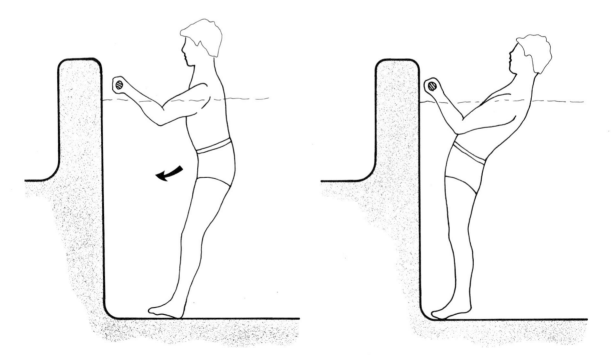

the hip joint and is particularly useful where the flexion deformity is minimal.

A quite different approach to applying stretch to fibrous tissue which is limiting joint movement is to use the momentum of the movement of a limb to produce a short duration stretch at the end of the movement which tries to carry the joint into the limited range.

Strengthening of weak muscle groups

It will depend largely upon which muscle groups are to be strengthened and their initial condition as to whether this is better carried out in the pool or in the physiotherapy department. The indications for strengthening exercise in the pool in this condition would be weak muscle groups where there is difficulty or discomfort maintaining a suitable starting position on dry land.

The exercises do not differ in principle to those used for strengthening muscle in the hydrotherapy treatment of any other condition, although modification may be necessary because of pain or severe limitation of movement. In such cases it is often useful to perform buoyancy resisted exercise, by choosing a float so large that the patient is unable to move it, and thus producing a static contraction.

Example. Resisted exercise to the hip extensors is required, but the patient finds that movement to the end of range extension produces pain. The patient is placed in the supine float support lying and a large float ring is placed under the foot. The patient is instructed to try to push the float down into the water. The buoyancy of the ring produces more resistance than the patient is able to overcome so that the hip extensors are working to their maximum but no movement takes place.

Re-education of function

It is common experience that those patients with osteoarthrosis of hips and knees for whom full weight-bearing on dry land is painful can often walk with little discomfort in the pool because of the reduction of body weight passing through the joint (see p. 121).

Even allowing for the differences in muscle work between weight-bearing in the pool and dry land walking, this is still a valuable treatment option, giving the opportunity to eliminate limps and other habits in the absence of pain.

The performing of many component movements of functional activities is often easier in the water when assisted by buoyancy, and the physiotherapist can take advantage of this in the early re-education of such movements. The practising of steps, standing and sitting are obvious examples, but time may usefully be spent on patients with stiff hips attempting movements associated with putting on socks, etc. Other activities will no doubt occur to the physiotherapist with patients having specific problems.

Associated joints

In the conservative treatment of osteoarthrosis the physiotherapist must remember that other joints may be involved secondarily to the joint which requires treatment. For example, in osteoarthrosis of the hip joint, the contralateral knee often becomes painful due to the abnormal strain which is placed upon it. Furthermore, where an osteoarthritic hip has very limited movement, a painful lumbar spine may develop because of abnormal compensatory movements in walking and in sitting. Where these problems have not arisen the physiotherapist should use some of the treatment time in strengthening quadriceps and in gentle mobilisation and strengthening of the lumbar spine as a preventative measure.

ANKYLOSING SPONDYLITIS

The use of hydrotherapy in this condition is probably not as common as it should be, bearing in mind that most patients could, after a short course of instruction in the pool, do their own exercises in their own time in the public swimming baths.

For many years this condition was regarded as a variant of rheumatoid arthritis and was sometimes known as rheumatoid arthritis of the spine. It is now more properly thought of as one part of a group of inter-related conditions among which are Crohn's disease, Whipple's disease, some forms of JCA and Behçet's syndrome. It is characterised by changes in the axial skeleton, which classically lead to ankylosis, and also to a more variable extent by the involvement of peripheral joints. The pathological changes occur as non-specific inflammation in the entheses (ligamentous attachments to bone), the synovium and the capsules. Eventually calcification of the spinal ligaments will occur and give rise to the typical deformities and resulting disabilities with which the physiotherapist will be familiar. Hydrotherapy will form only part of the total treatment programme of these patients and the aims of treatment will naturally be the same as those of the dry land physiotherapy:

a. The prevention and correction of deformity of the spine and other joints, mobilising, strengthening of extensor groups, relaxation of flexors and posture correction and re-education.

b. The maintenance and improvement of chest mobility and increase of vital capacity.

Some of these aims are more easily achieved in the hydrotherapy pool, whereas others are more appropriately tackled in the physiotherapy department or gymnasium.

As has been explained earlier (p. 60), entry into the pool and the consequent redistribution of body fluids cause an increase of venous return, and this represents approximately 700 ml increase of blood in the intrathoracic compartment (Lange et al 1974). This extra blood will decrease the potential vital capacity by the same amount. For the patient with ankylosing spondylitis with an already decreased vital capacity, this effect will be more significant than it would be to a normal person, but in practice rarely gives rise to problems. Patients with vital capacities as low as 30% of their predicted values have received pool treatment with no untoward effect (Harrison 1981). It should be remembered, however, that predicted values from normograms should be worked out using the patients' original height if this is reduced by the presence of a kyphus.

The patient may, however, feel some restriction in breathing on first entering the pool and he should be warned of this on his first visit. He should be told that the feeling, should it occur, will probably pass off quite quickly, but he should tell the therapist if he feels unwell.

Relaxation and stretching of flexor groups

It is in this aspect of the treatment that pool therapy is at its most useful in this condition. During recent years physiotherapists have become more aware of the fact that deformities in ankylosing spondylitis, which at first sight were fixed, could be improved considerably by the combined passive stretching and 'hold–relax' techniques (Bulstrode et al 1985). The use of this technique is especially effective since the warmth of the water and the general relaxation which it induces augments the results.

Hip flexors (Figs 8.3 and 8.4)

Flexion deformity of the hip joint, when some of this is due to shortening of the flexors rather than bony changes, is particularly responsive to this approach and serves to illustrate the method.

The patient stands facing the wall in the deeper part of the pool, holding the rail with an under hand grip, whilst keeping the trunk as close to the wall as his kyphus allows. This prevents the patient leaning forward, and goes some way to preventing unwanted movement in the other hip. If the patient is able, the opposite hip and knee may be fully flexed, the knee placed against the pool wall. This fixes the pelvis even more effectively. The hip being worked upon is extended with the knee straight, and the physiotherapist attaches a float to the foot or ankle. The size of the float will vary from patient to patient, but one with a buoyant upthrust of 2 kg will probably be required to produce the desired effect (p. 28).

The patient is then encouraged to relax and allow the float to carry the leg passively into extension. The patient should feel the float stretching the front of the hip joint, and if this is not the case then the float is not large enough and should be changed.

It is important that when floats are used in the manner described above, too large floats are not used or the movements may be difficult to control and the procedure becomes counter-productive.

When a point is reached where no further extension is being gained, the patient is instructed to pull the float down into the water a few inches and to hold this position. This contraction helps to gain a better relaxation of the flexors during the next relaxation period which follows after a few seconds, when the patient is told to relax and allow the float to stretch the hip again.

This is repeated several times until no increase in the range of movement is being gained.

Hip adductors

The patient stands side on to the wall of the pool holding on to the grab rail with both hands in order to hold the body close to the wall and fix the trunk (Fig. 8.5).

The procedure is the same as that used for the hip flexors. Floats are attached to the ankle and active buoyancy resisted contractions of the adductors are followed by twenty second periods of relaxation during which time the adductors are stretched passively.

Some of the movement gained in this way will obviously be lost after a few hours of normal everyday activities, but longer lasting improvement has been shown to be achieved if hip stretching is carried out regularly (Barefoot et al 1986).

Fig. 8.3 Starting position for stretching hip flexors by using floats

Fig. 8.4 Alternative position for stretching hip flexors by using floats

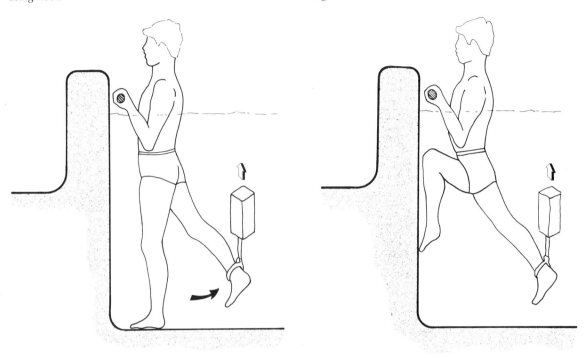

Fig. 8.5 Stretching hip adductors using floats

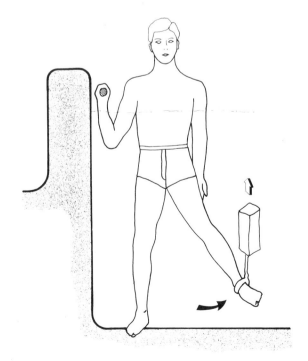

Underwater swimming

The spa resort of Leukerbad in Switzerland has for many years been treating ankylosing spondylitis patients by a physical treatment regime which includes underwater swimming.

The rationale for the inclusion of this activity is that since the patient must repeatly fill his lungs before diving, it is hoped that the vital capacity will be improved by the mobilisation of the costo-vertebral joints. If local conditions permit, e.g. size of pool, other patients, etc., some underwater swimming could be included in the treatment programme. Certainly it makes a useful activity with which to conclude an exercise session. The dangers, especially with patients who are very stiff, are obvious and the therapist should feel totally confident of her ability to cope with an emergency before embarking on this activity.

Recreational swimming

For many ankylosing spondylitis patients, membership of a disabled swimming club would be inappropriate, but they may be able to join a local branch of the National Ankylosing Spondylitis Society, many of which now organise pool sessions for their members.

Many patients, however, will prefer to make their own arrangements and make their trips to the local swimming pool into a family outing. It is important that such patients are taught 'home' exercises to do at their local pool as well as their 'dry land' exercise regime.

Group treatment (Fig. 8.6)

These patients are particularly well suited to hydrotherapy treatment in a group, because the same table of exercises can be applied to several patients with only minor modifications being made for individuals as the class progresses. It is essential that the physiotherapist, as always, has made a thorough assessment of each patient and made a mental note of their individual requirements and capabilities.

A second advantage of group treatment with these patients is that members motivate and encourage each other, and since they will be required to work hard, often with some discomfort, this results in a more effective treatment.

As with all class-taking the physiotherapist must be particularly alert for patients in difficulty. Correction of his loss of balance in the water is especially difficult for a patient with a rigid spine, and it is good practice when taking these classes for the therapist to position herself so that all the patients are in view the whole time. When the therapist finds it necessary to attend to an individual to assist or correct, then some of her attention must still be given to the rest of the group.

Neck movements

The neck may seem an unlikely part of the body to treat in the pool, but in this condition, where maintenance of cervical movement is so important, a few minutes of each session can usefully be given over to this end.

The patient stands in the deeper part of the pool with his back against the wall and, if necessary, with the knees bent so that the water just touches the chin. In this position the bulk of the trapezius muscle and the long neck muscles are immersed in the warm water and this helps to induce their relaxation.

Movements of rotation and side flexion are then carried out as free exercise. If there is limitation, more movement can often be gained by static self-resisted exercise in which the patient places his palm on the side of his face and resists the movement. Static work is then alternated with active movement as the range is gradually increased.

Fig. 8.6 An ankylosing spondylitis pool class

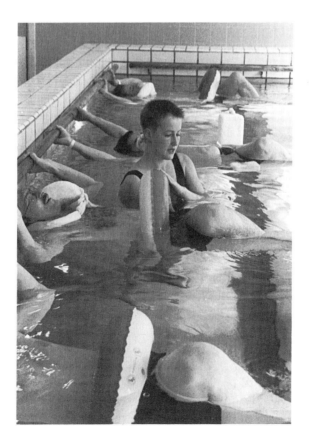

RHEUMATOID ARTHRITIS   In Britain alone one and a half million people suffer from this condition, so the chances are that all hydrotherapy departments will have such patients attending for treatment.

There is much evidence to support the idea that this is not a single disease, but is more properly regarded as a syndrome consisting of:

1. Progressive inflammatory polyarthritis of peripheral joints
2. Positive rheumatoid factor
3. Marginal erosions around the affected joints.

Foremost in the physiotherapist's mind when treating these patients will be the pathological changes which occur in the joints, for it is the physical effects which these changes produce and the functional deficit produced by these effects, at which the physical treatment is aimed.

It should constantly be borne in mind, however, that although the condition is named arthritis after its most obvious clinical signs, many organs and tissues are involved and there is often metabolic disturbance due to the disease processes. The patient may be febrile, anaemic, underweight and feel generally unwell, and this may sometimes vary from treatment to treatment. These general considerations will dictate the type and the duration of the exercise treatment programme.

Rheumatoid arthritis is probably the condition most associated with treatment by hydrotherapy, and it would be difficult to imagine a patient with this condition where pool therapy could not usefully form part of the total treatment programme.

The main aim in the treatment of this condition should, however, as with any other physical treatment, be the measurable improvement in some physical parameter which has been chosen after a thorough assessment of the patient's condition and needs.

In rheumatoid arthritis the ability of the patient to perform exercises which will achieve these aims is aided by the warmth of the water, which eases pain and gives the subjective feeling of being less stiff. The ease with which patients are able to perform movements in the pool, as opposed to dry land, is occasionally something from which the physiotherapist must protect the patient. There is always the temptation for an enthusiastic patient to do too much, too quickly. This is especially the case with patients who have not had pool treatment before and over-indulge their new found freedom of movement.

The patient who is referred for treatment is better assessed in the physiotherapy department, and a whole session may be set aside for this if the patient is new to the department.

Patients will often appreciate a treatment early in the day since pool treatment helps many patients to get rid of their morning stiffness more easily. This must, however, be weighed against the fact that getting themselves ready for treatment before their morning stiffness has started to ease off may be too difficult.

Occasionally, when a patient is attending as an out-patient and suffers a 'flare up', it may be appropriate to suspend treatment for a while until things have settled down. Not only will the patient be unable to perform the exercise programme, but the rigours of the journey and the handling will probably nullify any benefit the patient might gain from the relief of pain and stiffness as a result of the warm water.

Strengthening exercises

In the severe rheumatoid patient, gross muscle wasting is not an uncommon finding, and the pool is particularly useful in the early stages of muscle strengthening. The relatively small resistances required are easily provided, and whereas it is often difficult to make the patient comfortable in a suitable starting position on a treatment couch, in the pool there is usually no problem. The patient can be placed in buoyancy support lying and the warmth of the water contributes to pain relief.

Since the joints in rheumatoid arthritis are often unstable one must be careful, on giving resisted exercises, that strain is not placed upon the joint over which the muscle being strengthened is working or any other joint.

This calls for advance planning and for constant modification of strengthening exercises to suit each individual joint's requirements if damage is to be avoided. Measures which may be used to modify strengthening exercises to prevent strain on ligaments are:
1. Manual support to the joint during the exercise
2. Selection of a starting position such that a resisted static contraction is performed where this will render the joint less vulnerable to strain
3. Limiting the movement during the exercise to a small range where there is least chance of damaging the joint
4. Splinting of joints which may be at risk during strengthening.

With these patients the physiotherapist may not always be aiming to strengthen muscles to their physiological normal, since the degree of muscle strength required will be determined by the amount of activity which the state of the joints will allow.

All the methods which can be used in hydrotherapy for muscle strengthening may be used on these patients provided that the precautions already mentioned are taken.

Mobilisation of stiff joints

It is in this area of treatment that the physiotherapist working with rheumatoid patients must take particular care, for insensitive treatment may result in the joint becoming more painful.

The gentle stretching of the fibrous tissue which is limiting movement must be carried out in a controlled manner, in which the stretching can be increased by small increments. The physiotherapist should relate the rate of progression of the mobilising to the 'feed back' obtained from the patient. The patient's report on the effects of the last treatment should be compared with her records of the last treatment and suitable adjustments made.

Obviously, if fibrous tissue is to be stretched then there will be some discomfort after treatment, but this should not last for more than twelve hours or so, and if the patient is experiencing discomfort after twenty-four hours then the treatment was too intensive and should be modified.

A rheumatoid joint which is painful and limited in its range of movement will almost certainly be limited to some extent by tight muscle, and all attempts to mobilise by stretching adhesions should be preceded by exercise to relax the muscles working over that joint. The usual way to mobilise these joints is by free unresisted exercise performed initially well within the patient's range. When the muscles are relaxed the patient is encouraged gradually to increase the range until he is giving a gentle stretch at the end of range. The buoyancy supported position is more commonly used in this type of exercise, but buoyancy assisted exercise may be employed. It is probably not advisable, however, to increase the buoyancy of the limb by using floats. If the assistance from buoyancy is minimal, unguarded movements are less likely to occur.

Use of Bad Ragaz techniques

There is sometimes reluctance to use these techniques with rheumatoid patients because the exercises are mistakenly thought to be too vigorous.

One must remember that in most Bad Ragaz patterns the resistance produced is, in fact, determined by the patient and is directly proportional to the amount of effort the patient expends. Probably more important is the possibility that the joints may be overstretched or that the ligaments may be subjected to strain which is likely to damage them. Both of these possibilities are totally avoidable and should certainly not be regarded as contra-indicating this approach if other considerations suggest its use.

'Overstretching'

The danger of this happening is likely to arise where a movement is brought to an end by the joint reaching its end of range and where that range is limited by fibrous adhesion.

Example. When treating a patient with weak quadriceps muscle it may be appropriate to use the Bad Ragaz technique of single hip and knee extension as illustrated in Figures 6.15 and 6.16.

The resistance provided by the water in this exercise is small and consequently the patient will move away from the physiotherapist quite quickly. As has already been suggested, the momentum which is gained in such movements may be used to stretch a joint where this is appropriate, but joints having inflammatory joint disease must be protected from such uncontrolled stretching.

This effect can be avoided if the patient is instructed to relax just before the end of range is reached. Alternatively, the physiotherapist may push the foot away from herself, i.e. put the knee into flexion just before full extension is reached.

Strain on ligaments

This will occur where counter-pressure to resisted movement is applied to the patient's limb in an injudicious way. It happens most often when there is a joint between the pivot of the movement and the point of application of the resistance. It will be seen, therefore, that the most likely joints to be affected by this are the elbow or wrist when the shoulder muscles are being resisted or the knee joint when the hip muscles are being resisted.

Example. When resisted ab- and adduction of the hip is being carried out the co-lateral ligaments of the knee will be compromised if counter-pressure is applied distal to the knee joint and no provision is made to support the knee joint from lateral movements. See Figure 6.23.

Protective splints

It is not unusual for one joint to be inflamed whilst the rest of the patient's joints are relatively quiescent. More often than not in such cases, it is sufficient to leave that particular joint out of the exercise programme, but on occasion it may be necessary to immobilise it, especially if it is very painful. Temporary splints for use in the hydrotherapy pool can be made of Plastazote; the commonest joints to be splinted in this way are the knee and elbow.

A large percentage of rheumatoid patients have neck involvement to a greater or lesser degree and the wearing of flotation collars in the hydrotherapy pool often provokes neck pain or discomfort. This can usually be prevented by making Plastazote collars for the patients which they wear beneath their flotation collars.

Aspiration and intra-articular injections

Patients frequently have one or more of their joints aspirated and it is not uncommon for a mixture of steroid and local anaesthetic to be injected at the same time.

It has become generally accepted practice to allow 24 hours to elapse after such a procedure before pool therapy is continued.

Handling of patients (Fig. 8.7)

For a severe rheumatoid patient, a hydrotherapy treatment will involve being lifted and handled. The patient will need help to put on his bathing costume, move from chair to hoist and so on. It is important that unqualified staff appreciate that when lifting and handling rheumatoid patients there are particular points to bear in mind over and above the general principles they have been taught.

Painful joints

The technique of lifting should not place strain on the rheumatoid joint and periarticular structures. Shoulder joints are particularly vulnerable, and it is better to avoid underarm lifting where possible. Fixed flexion deformities of the knees should always be supported and the lifting points should not be such that they tend to straighten the knee.

It is always worthwhile asking such patients how they prefer to be lifted, and if this does not put the patient or the helpers at risk then this should be the method of choice.

Manipulating damp arms into dressing-gown sleeves can be painful to those patients with shoulder involvement and should be avoided if possible. In departments where many rheumatoid or other disabled patients are treated, it may be worth considering making some poncho style pool gowns which can be slipped over the patients' heads (see p. 33).

Fig. 8.7 Rheumatoid patient being received into the pool from the hoist

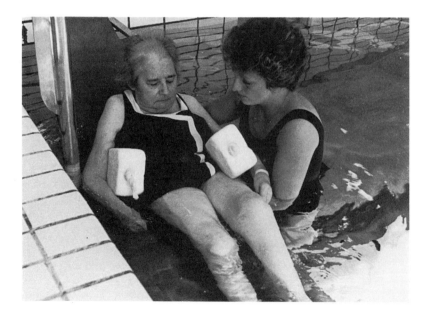

Poor skin

Many patients with rheumatoid arthritis, and particularly those who are, or have been, on steroid therapy, have thin 'tissue-paper' skin, which is usually most marked on the forearms and the shins. Great care must be taken when handling these patients who should never be gripped, but supported on the helpers' palms or forearms. Patients of this sort are very vulnerable when their bathing costumes are being pulled over their shins, and helpers should be particularly warned of this.

FRACTURES

Fractures of the lower limb

Treatment of these patients in the hydrotherapy pool will be aimed at the direct results of the fracture and at the secondary results of immobilisation. Any external fixation will have been removed and wounds will have largely healed before treatment takes place.

The aims of the treatment will be:
1. Mobilisation of joints which are stiff due to immobilisation or to damage at the time of the fracture
2. Strengthening of atrophied muscle
3. Re-education of function, the most important of which will be walking, stairs, standing and sitting.

Mobilisation

Where it is required to increase the range of movement of joints which have become stiff through immobilisation, exercises which give an overstretch at the end of the movement should be used, since the aim is to stretch the fibrous adhesions which have formed in the capsule of the joint and its periarticular structures.

These exercises should not necessarily be limited by discomfort, but the patient should be warned that after the treatment the joint may ache and that this is an indication that the treatment is having the desired effect. This assumes that the fracture site is sound, but where this is not the case the physiotherapist should remember that the lever is a powerful machine and mobilisation of a joint in the proximity of an unsound fracture site may result in damage.

Given that the fracture is united, mobilisation with these patients will proceed at a quicker pace than those with joint disease.

The patient should be told the measurements which are obtained from goniometry, targets should be set and the joint should be measured at suitable intervals and the results used to encourage the patient to further effort. Techniques for mobilising stiff joints will be the same as those used in any other condition where there is no inflammatory joint disease (see p. 145). The joint in the lower limb which is most likely to require such treatment is the knee joint. If the knee has been immobilised in the extended position, there will often be very little movement when the external fixation is removed and this is invariably the case where the knee joint has suffered some trauma at the time of the fracture. In such cases the later results of swelling and its organisation will add to the limitation of movement which is brought by adhesions in muscle tissue and of periarticular structures.

When flexion is minimal (say less than 15 degrees), exercise in the pool is probably not the best way of increasing range of movement since such exercises depend upon momentum providing the force necessary to stretch fibrous tissue. If the amount of movement is small, then it is difficult to obtain sufficient momentum to provide adequate stretch.

This illustrates one of the difficulties which often arises during the mobilisation of joints in the hydrotherapy pool, i.e. the problem of gaining adequate fixation so that the movement may be accurately localised to the joint being treated. It is often a help in this case to put the patient on the pool plinth or stool which then gives the patient something solid to work against.

Since the pool will be used for strengthening and partial weight-bearing, some mobilisation can be achieved even when joint range is minimal, but it is probably better at this early stage to supplement this with mobilising exercises in the physiotherapy department.

All the various methods of mobilising in the pool can be used on these joints and it is useful to do so since the treatment can become tedious for the patient if only one or two exercises are used.

The programme can, therefore, include free exercises, exercises using floats as passive stretching agents and Bad Ragaz patterns which can give overstretch at the end of range as well as activities which will tend to increase the range of movement.

Facilities for undercurrent douche will not exist in many departments, but where they do this will be a useful preparation for these exercises. This is a jet of water, slightly warmer than the pool which can be played around the joint to have a similar effect to 'finger kneading' (see p. 174).

Strengthening of muscle

With most of these patients the physiotherapist will be hoping to achieve, at the end of the final treatment, a muscle which is of normal strength. Bearing in mind that in fractures of the lower limb, the muscles concerned are most probably the quadriceps and the hip extensors, the pool will not be appropriate for the final stages of strengthening where large loads will be necessary to be effective. It is visualised that treatment in the physiotherapy department will be carried out in parallel with the hydrotherapy, and that as the muscles pass from the early to middle stage the accent on this aspect of the treatment will fall on the 'dry land' physiotherapy.

The physiotherapist may choose to load the muscles to be strengthened by the use of floats for buoyancy resisted exercises or to use the Bad Ragaz techniques described in Chapter 6. The treatment may include both these techniques, but whatever method is chosen the physiotherapist must remember that in order to strengthen muscle it must be worked to its maximum and there will be a point when most pool strengthening exercise will no longer fulfil this requirement. The physiotherapist must make suitable changes in the treatment programme immediately this point is reached or valuable treatment time will be wasted.

Re-education of function

Walking

Many patients who have fractures of the lower limbs are often anxious and apprehensive when the time for partial weight-bearing arrives and are reluctant to put weight through the limb.

Pool treatment is extremely useful at this stage and most patients will soon gain confidence in their leg's ability to weight-bear. A preliminary exercise which will encourage the patient to put weight through the limb, can be performed before the patient is actually put into the standing position.

Example. The patient is supported in floats in the supine lying position and pushed towards the side of the pool, so that the feet are against the wall and the knees bent as in Figure 8.8.

The patient is then told to push himself away from the wall using both feet whilst the physiotherapist moves backwards to give room for the movement and to catch the patient after the 'push'.

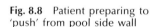

Fig. 8.8 Patient preparing to 'push' from pool side wall

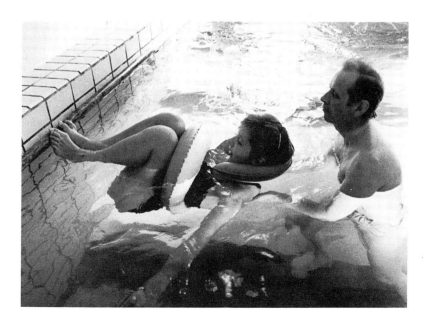

When it is apparent to the physiotherapist that the patient is using the affected leg, then the exercise may be progressed by asking the patient to use only this leg for pushing off, the other knee being flexed to keep it out of the way. This type of exercise will probably give the patient confidence more quickly than placing him on his feet straight away. There are, of course, patients where the difficulty is not that of encouraging them to put weight through the limb, but rather of preventing them from weight-bearing too heavily. Where minimal weight-bearing is indicated and the patient has difficulty comprehending the instructions regarding the amount of weight to put through the limb, the pool offers a solution.

The degree of immersion of the patient will determine the amount of weight passing through the lower limbs quite independently of the patient's will, and the physiotherapist can be certain of the percentage weight-bearing which is taking place.

The rationale behind the progression of weight-bearing in the pool and methods by which it may be applied are given in Chapter 7.

Fractures of the upper limb

Fractures of the upper limb are not commonly treated by hydrotherapy, and in some departments they are never treated in this way. Certainly there would be little to justify treating fractures of the wrist and forearm in the pool, but for fractures of the humerus, which invariably result in loss of movement at the shoulder joint, pool therapy is an excellent mode of treatment.

This is particularly the case with impacted fractures of the surgical neck of the humerus where early movement is indicated. This early movement is uncomfortable and the patient is often apprehensive to start moving his shoulder so quickly after the fracture. These patients can begin pool therapy after a few days and the warmth of the water and the buoyant support make this treatment more tolerable than dry land mobilising exercises.

The patient can enter the pool wearing a sling and need not remove it until seated in the pool with the arm fully submerged. The seat should be of such a height that the water comes just above the level of the tip of the shoulder, and it is in this position that the exercises will be given in the early stages of treatment.

This position is difficult for some patients to maintain unless they are able to grip the sides of the seat with both hands. This is because the weight holding them is almost countered by the buoyant upthrust when immersed to this level (see p. 121). The physiotherapist must, therefore, hold the patient down onto the seat and anticipate this difficulty rather than waiting until it arises or the patient's confidence will be lost. This can be done by the physiotherapist kneeling behind the patient and holding the hips, or she can kneel in front of the patient and hold the patient's thighs down on to the seat. With these patients it is probably better, at least initially, to be in front of the patient since it gives the patient confidence and also gives the physiotherapist the opportunity to see the patient's face and judge the amount of discomfort produced by the exercises (see Fig. 8.9).

The early treatments will consist of buoyancy assisted movements of flexion, extension and abduction, at first only within the range of comfort, and this will gradually gain relaxation of the adductor muscles and the range may then be increased.

From the outset it will be necessary to correct reversed humeroscapular rhythm which is invariably introduced unconsciously into the movement by the patient. It is in this aspect that the treatment in the pool has a disadvantage over dry land treatment, since it is not possible to demonstrate this incorrect movement to the patient by using a mirror. The physiotherapist can, however, demonstrate the movements by performing them herself so that the patient understands what is required.

Later, as more movement is gained and the discomfort becomes less, free exercises in the buoyancy supporting position may be introduced. Gradually, resisted exercise using float or bats can be used, aiming at increasing the strength of the abductors of the shoulders which will have lost muscle bulk as a result of disuse.

The patient will have been taught exercises for home use which will include rotation both medial and lateral, and in the final stages the Bad Ragaz arm patterns will be useful for final strengthening and also to gain any rotation which is still lacking.

Fig. 8.9 Sitting position for shoulder exercises

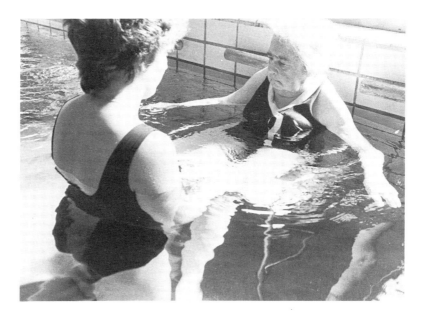

BACK CONDITIONS

The hydrotherapy pool is a very useful treatment medium for patients with generalised lack of spinal mobility such as follows trauma to the vertebral column including fractures and also following surgery, in particular laminectomy.

Fractures of the vertebrae

Fractures of the vertebrae occur usually following direct local trauma or due to a compressive force on the vertebral bodies as would occur if the patient had fallen from a height. Wedge fractures of the vertebral bodies and fractures of the transverse processes are essentially stable and no neurological signs result. However, these patients will experience pain and discomfort and a period of bed rest for one to four weeks is usually necessary. Following this, a programme of mobilising and strengthening exercises is commenced in the pool and on dry land and the patient is encouraged to mobilise within the limits of his pain.

Patients with unstable fractures, even without neurological signs, will be kept on a longer period of bed rest until the fracture is stable. Once this has occurred the patient begins a mobilising and strengthening programme as for patients with stable fractures, although it will probably be necessary to progress this more slowly.

Fracture dislocations of the vertebrae with compression, torsion or kinking of the spinal cord will result in paralysis of muscles and other neurological signs below the level of the lesion. Pool therapy for this group of patients is described later in this chapter (p. 164).

Laminectomy

This is a surgical procedure in which the laminae (either one or both) of a vertebrae or several vertebrae are removed. This is done to relieve pressure on the spinal cord such as results from a herniated disc, or to remove a tumour.

The incision is in the midline, the vertebral muscles are stripped back and the appropriate laminae removed. The offending disc or tumour is thus exposed and excised.

Following surgery, a post-operative regime of mobilisation will be commenced. Surgeons differ very much in their ideas on how quickly a patient should be mobilised and to what extent flexion is to be included in the regime. Clearly, account must be taken of the surgeon's wishes and the exercise programme structured accordingly.

Treatment

Water is an ideal medium in which to commence mobilising the spine following injury and surgery. The range of movement permitted can be easily controlled and strengthening exercises progressed in the supportive medium of warm water. Gait re-education and standing activities are very useful and can usually be progressed fairly quickly.

In the early stages, care must be taken to ensure comfortable positioning of the body supporting ring. It is sometimes more easy to use a linen or nylon sling with Plastazote or cork floats, as these are easier to slip under the patient. Patterns of movement for the lower extremities and trunk using the Bad Ragaz method are ideal and can be done slowly through a small part of range until the patient's confidence and a decrease in pain permit larger movements.

It is a good idea to commence with bilateral abduction and adduction patterns as symmetry of the body in relation to the water is maintained; the tendency to roll will be minimised, and by the muscle activity in the legs irradiation will occur into the trunk muscles. Reinforcement can be put into the trunk extensors or flexors by emphasising either extension or flexion respectively in the hip component.

Trunk patterns in supine with pelvic or upper or lower extremity fixation can be gently encouraged and progressed to vigorous full range movements (Fig. 8.10).

Standing balance with stabilising activity can be reinforced by creating areas of turbulence in front, behind and to the sides of the patient as he stands in water as deep as possible. Walking forwards and then backwards with rapid reversal of direction also, with the patient keeping his arms straight holding 'table tennis bat' paddles, are some other activities which can be given to these patients in the water.

Fig. 8.10 Trunk side flexion exercise, using a half-plinth to fix upper trunk

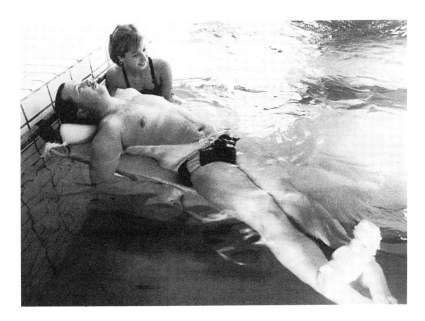

NEUROLOGICAL CONDITIONS

CONDITIONS RESULTING IN HYPOTONUS AND FLACCID PARALYSIS

This group of conditions includes anterior poliomyelitis, polyneuropathy, Guillain-Barré syndrome and muscular dystrophies.

The pathological signs and symptoms of these conditions are briefly described, but the reader is referred to other texts for fuller descriptions.

Polyneuropathy

The exact cause of a polyneuropathy is not always known, although the causative factor is often toxic or metabolic.

The first symptoms which the patient experiences are frequently those of numbness or tingling in the hands and feet. These may be accompanied by motor signs of weakness in the distal muscles. The sensory and motor signs and symptoms extend upwards to involve more proximal muscles of hips, shoulder girdle and, in the more severe cases, the trunk and respiratory muscles. No spasticity or increase in muscle tone which characterises involvement of the upper motor neurone occurs. The muscle weakness is flaccid and there is a decrease in tone. The reflexes are diminished or absent and the sensory changes are often described as 'glove and stocking anaesthesia'. If the respiratory muscles are involved to any great extent, it will be necessary to perform a tracheostomy and to ventilate the patient artificially.

There is a tremendous variation in the extent to which sensory and motor changes occur. Some patients will experience only minor sensory involvement and slight weakness in distal muscle groups, whilst others will be totally paralysed, requiring artificial ventilation. After a short time, one to three weeks when the signs and symptoms are at their maximum, the motor paralysis improves slowly and the patient can commence active rehabilitation.

Guillain-Barré syndrome

This is a condition sometimes described as infective polyneuritis, which very much resembles the description of a toxic or metabolic polyneuropathy given above. However, this disease usually develops following some kind of non-specific pyrexial illness which the patient experienced during the preceding weeks. The onset is similar, as is the progress of the disease, to polyneuropathy. Very often these patients do require artificial ventilation and it is not uncommon to find cranial nerve involvement as well as peripheral. Full recovery frequently occurs, but may take as long as eighteen months to two years.

Anterior poliomyelitis

This condition is caused by a virus which attacks the anterior horn cells, in the more severe cases resulting in a flaccid paralysis of varying degree and distribution. Occasionally the cranial nuclei are affected causing a bulbar paralysis. The majority of cases of poliomyelitis do not progress to the paralytic stage, symptoms being confined to pyrexia, headache, intestinal upset, neck stiffness and aching in the muscles of the back and thighs in particular.

In western countries this disease is only very infrequently seen due to extensive use of the oral vaccine. However, the physiotherapist who works in the Third World will find that this disease and its consequences contribute very considerably to her workload.

Treatment

Common to all the above conditions, any paralysis if it develops will be flaccid in nature. In describing pool therapy for these conditions, all will be discussed together from the early stages to late rehabilitation, assuming a paralytic state has developed.

Pool therapy can be commenced as soon as the medical staff are satisfied that the patient is no longer febrile and, in the case of poliomyelitis, no longer infectious. It is unwise to be over-ambitious and to take the patient who still has an open tracheostomy into the pool, although this is occasionally done, but clearly with particular care being taken. Apart from these precautions the earlier the severely paralysed patient is taken into the pool the better.

The patient can be put into swimming trunks in the ward at the time when the nurses are attending to him. If possible he should be brought to the hydrotherapy department in his bed as this reduces the number of times he must be transferred and is thus less fatiguing for both patient and staff.

In the department, the patient is transferred onto the stretcher which is attachable to the hoist. The patient is wheeled on the stretcher to the shower and the patient showered with the water temperature at 37 °C. The stretcher is then attached to the hoist and lowered into the pool. There must be at least one physiotherapist in the pool to receive the patient. As the patient enters the water, the physiotherapist must be at his head end and support him under the thorax, floating him off the stretcher. For the first treatment session, if space allows, it is advisable to leave the stretcher in the water so that if necessary the patient can be taken out quickly.

Whilst the physiotherapist is supporting the patient at the thorax, with his head on her shoulder, a second physiotherapist places a large body ring over the patient's feet and legs to position it at the pelvis. Alternatively, a buoyant sling float is positioned at the pelvis if this is easier and providing it gives enough support. A small ring can be placed around each ankle or one around both ankles if there is a tendency for the flail lower extremities to move in the water out of control. Depending upon the degree of confidence of the patient (and also of the physiotherapist), an inflatable horse-shoe shaped neck collar can be positioned under the patient's neck and thus he can float free in the water supported by rings. If the patient is anxious, this is better left to a later treatment session by which time he will be more confident and used to the water.

With these severely paralysed patients it should again be emphasised that the manual holds or contacts should be proximal on the patient, particularly in the early hydrotherapy sessions.

Following the detailed examination of the patient on dry land, which amongst other findings will indicate the muscle groups involved, a treatment plan specific to the hydrotherapy sessions must be evolved.

As it is likely that all major muscle groups of the extremities and trunk will be affected, the pool session should commence with the stronger uninvolved or less involved muscle groups being worked. Usually this will indicate the trunk muscles. In the event of total, apparently equal involvement of all extremity and trunk muscles, then again work should commence with the trunk as being the most proximal area.

Whilst in the pool, it will be found most valuable to exercise the patient in the supine and side-lying positions in the early stages. Sitting with the water to the level of the shoulders to do arm activities, is not easy for the patient. Not only is it difficult for him to have any stability in the sitting position, but also the hydrostatic pressure on the thorax can embarrass respiration. Until he has good sitting balance on dry land, arm activities are best done in supine lying. It is not of any value to have the patient upright for walking activities with his legs splinted if he does not have sufficient strength in the trunk muscles to maintain an upright posture.

Exercises for trunk strengthening using the Bad Ragaz method are particularly valuable.

With manual contacts on the posterior chest wall, trunk side flexion can be given with slow movements. Rotation of the trunk is encouraged by the physiotherapist turning the upper trunk very slightly in one direction and asking the patient to try to follow with the pelvis.

As muscle strength increases, larger although still slow, movements are used and the patient progresses to trunk flexion and extension in supine.

For early, lower extremity work, bilateral abduction and adduction patterns with flexion, extension and rotation components are given. It is very likely that in the early stages it will be necessary for the physiotherapist to use her manual contacts more proximally and to place her hands on the appropriate aspects of the lower thighs, just proximal to or at the knees. It is advantageous in the early stages to use movement patterns, i.e. isotonic work rather than stabilising work, as it is easier for such a patient to organise his muscle activity to move rather than to hold. The ability to stabilise is, of course, vital for normal posture and movement and therefore isometric work should be added as early as possible.

Pool activity and specific exercises are progressed as the patient gains in strength. The Bad Ragaz or ring method can be used most advantageously with these patients, as the water can be used to assist or resist movement; general handling of the paralysed patient is safe and easy and the patient benefits psychologically as he achieves even the smallest activity in water which would be very difficult on dry land. As recovery and increase in strength occur, patterns of movement, with manual contacts to emphasise finer areas of muscle work, i.e. dorsi and plantar flexion of the feet, inversion and eversion, can be reinforced from the stronger proximal muscle groups.

Standing activities and gait re-education are added to the programme as early as possible, if necessary with the use of weighted sandals and Plastazote leg splints.

Hydrotherapy contributes greatly to the rehabilitation programme of these patients, but it must always be remembered that exercises in the medium of warm water does put a greater demand on the cardiovascular and respiratory systems, than the same amount of exercise on dry land. Therefore, it is vital that these patients do not become fatigued. Sessions should be short, possibly starting with five minutes and progressing in length only as the patient's general condition allows. These patients do require at least one hour of rest following a hydrotherapy session, and the patient's day programme must be scheduled accordingly. It should, however, be realistic to expect to treat the patient in the pool daily.

Muscular dystrophies

These are a group of progressive disorders involving degeneration of certain groups of muscles. Onset occurs usually during the first ten years of life and is characterised by symmetrical muscle weakness.

In the pseudohypertrophic type, although muscle groups appear to be enlarged, weakness as in the other types is also the predominant sign.

The prognosis for patients suffering from any of the muscular dystrophies is poor, with life expectancy seldom extending beyond early middle age. In the pseudohypertrophic type, death usually occurs when the patient is in his teens. It is very uncommon for a female to be affected.

Treatment of any nature does not appear to have any influence on the course of the disease. Maintaining mobility and independence for as long as possible is, therefore, of importance both from the physical and psychological point of view.

Treatment

As this group of diseases is progressive in nature and the prognosis poor, it must be accepted that no physical improvement can be expected by a period of hydrotherapy, nor by any other physical means. Indeed, some patients become so fatigued after a pool session, that this mode of treatment is contra-indicated.

However, the majority of patients with this condition benefit enormously from the opportunity to move in the medium of water and to perform activities which are not possible for them on dry land. The pool session is, therefore, largely related to general activity, including swimming without too much emphasis being placed on any particular group of muscles. It is particularly important with these patients to ascertain whether there was any undue fatigue following the previous hydrotherapy session and to adjust the activities and time spent in the pool accordingly. A rest period following the pool session is also of value for these patients. Perhaps the greatest benefit of hydrotherapy for these patients is psychological in nature and this can be enhanced by group treatment in the water, particularly for children.

SPINAL CORD LESIONS

Lesions of the spinal cord can occur as a result of trauma or of a specific pathology, with a resultant loss of sensation, motor power and autonomic control below the level of the lesion. There may be complete loss in all these areas or only partial, resulting in an incomplete para or tetraplegia. The paralysis may be entirely flaccid or there may be varying degrees of spasticity in the extremities.

Spina bifida

During development of the fetus the vertebral canal fails to close and in addition there is usually an associated abnormality of the spinal cord. In its most severe form, a sac containing meninges and possibly also the spinal cord protrudes through the defect in the spinal column: this is known as a meningomyelocele. Hydrocephalus is a common associated abnormality. There is a resultant loss of sensation and motor power in the lower limbs and trunk (depending upon the level of the spinal abnormality) and paralysis of the sphincters. If hydrocephalus is present there may also be a mental defect. In the less severe forms, where there is only a structural defect in the vertebrae without protrusion, there will be few, if any, signs and symptoms to detect clinically, the diagnosis being made by radiological examination.

Treatment of spinal cord lesions, including spina bifida

Children and adults with these conditions which result in paraplegia or tetraplegia should be taken into the pool as early as possible. Apart from the therapeutic value, for the rest of their lives water will provide an ideal medium for recreation and competitive sport in whatever part of the country they live. Therefore, helping the patient to overcome any anxiety in early pool sessions is of great benefit in the long term as well as for any treatment purposes.

Some patients show signs of hypertonus in the affected extremities and these should be counteracted as far as possible, particularly in the early stages after injury. However, those patients who have to contend with spasticity should not be precluded from swimming and other similar activities, and should be encouraged to participate.

Whilst the causes of spinal cord lesions vary, the disabilities resulting are similar and, therefore, for purposes of describing a hydrotherapy programme for these patients, they will be described as one. Differentiation, however, needs to be made between those patients who present with a complete spinal cord lesion and those with an incomplete lesion.

Incomplete spinal cord lesion

Patients who have an irregular distribution of active movement remaining in various muscle groups of an extremity or trunk require very specific treatment in order to fully potentiate all remaining muscle activity. Care must be taken not to increase spasticity and this can usually be done by altering the patient's starting position, i.e. perhaps in side-lying rather than in supine and by breaking up a pattern of movement. For instance, if working on the hip extensors the knee should be kept in flexion to prevent the full extensor pattern occurring. To prevent any sudden movements which may result in an increase in spasticity the patient should be supported by rings and floats, and particular care must be taken to prevent any other patient or therapist colliding with the patient.

Trunk work is extremely important for these patients and all patterns should be used for strengthening and mobilising. Upper extremities also should be fully worked, with special attention being given to the muscle groups of the shoulder girdle and to latissimus dorsi in particular.

Maximum use must be made of irradiation, the proximal muscle groups of normal innervation being used to irradiate to the more distal weaker groups. Standing and walking activities may or may not be realistic and this must be assessed with the physiotherapist and others who are treating the patient on dry land. If appropriate, gait activities may require the use of back splints for one or both legs and possibly weighted sandals for the feet.

Once the patient's autonomic system is stable and he has fully adjusted to the water and working in the humid atmosphere, the patient should have little problem with fatigue and the physiotherapist can usually increase time in the hydrotherapy pool to half hour periods very quickly. It is, however, recommended that these patients only be treated for five to ten minutes on the first occasion to ensure that no untoward effect results.

Complete spinal cord lesions

Hydrotherapy for these patients is used to assist the patient to build up all available muscle groups. As such, it is most useful in the early stages of mobilising, but much stronger muscle work in the nature of weight and pulley systems and multigym use should be given as strength increases in the physiotherapy department.

In the pool, upper extremity and trunk work is given with maximal resistance. The patient can work from the supine and side-lying positions and, as he becomes more adjusted to the water, the prone position can be encouraged.

Most particularly for these patients, swimming should be encouraged, the early strokes and adjustments being learnt in the hydrotherapy pool before progression to a normal swimming pool. In the water the patient can be taught a variety of activities such as somersaults and underwater swimming which encourage him to become fully confident in the medium.

CONDITIONS RESULTING IN HYPERTONUS

Hypertonus or spasticity occur in many conditions where the lesion involves the cerebral cortex and upper motor neurones. The most usual conditions with which patients are referred for pool therapy or for which it is felt pool therapy could be helpful include:
— Hemiplegia
— Head injury
— Multiple sclerosis.

Compared with conditions resulting in hypotonus, pool therapy is more limited in its effectiveness where spasticity is a predominating sign. However, certain specific activities can, for some patients, be advantageously worked on in the medium of water.

One of the greatest disadvantages of the use of water as an exercise medium for patients with spasticity is the fact that there is no stable support on which the patient lies. He can, of course, be supported in the water by buoyant apparatus and, therefore, particularly if in the supine position, will be in relative equilibrium. As there is no firm underlying support it is very difficult to inhibit pathological patterns of movement while facilitating the normal. In handling patients with hypertonus it is important that no activity is allowed to reinforce abnormal patterns and cause associated reactions.

However, particularly with children, use of the head, either to facilitate rolling or to work against the tendency of the asymmetrical body to roll, can be encouraged to advantage.

Swimming is a beneficial recreational activity for many in these groups of conditions and in the authors' opinion can best be taught by the Halliwick method.

Hemiplegia

Hemiplegia may occur following a cerebral thrombosis, embolism or haemorrhage. A tumour lying in one of the cerebral hemispheres or trauma to one hemisphere can also result in hemiplegia. Loss of consciousness is not unusual following a cerebral vascular accident: this may be transient or last for a longer period of time. Initially, there is usually hypotonus, but as the period of cerebral shock and the oedema subsides, hypertonus may become evident. As well as spasticity, diminished proprioception and possible hemianopia are significant factors which can delay rehabilitation if they are not recognised.

Head injuries

Head injuries which occur as a result of trauma (most usually road traffic accidents) can cause signs and symptoms which vary very considerably in their severity and distribution. A patient may only be slightly dazed and show no signs of physical or mental impairment. At the other extreme, there may be loss of consciousness over a long period of time, gross physical problems and behavioural changes, the patient after a long period of rehabilitation requiring continuing care.

Of all the various signs and symptoms which may occur in the more severely affected, spasticity, rigidity and ataxia are those most commonly found.

Multiple sclerosis

The cause of multiple sclerosis remains unknown. It manifests itself by patchy demyelination of the white matter of the nervous system. The disease is characterised by periods of exacerbation and remission. In some patients the course of the disease is very rapid—death can occur as soon as three months after onset. In other cases, the disease progresses very slowly with long periods of remission.

Early symptoms which occur include optic neuritis, double vision, numbness of part of the body, usually a limb, weakness, especially the dragging of a foot, and disturbance of micturition. Females in early adulthood are most commonly affected. As the disease progresses, paraparesis usually develops, together with sensory loss. Spasticity further develops with weakness in the upper extremities and decreasing vision, severely limiting the patient's level of function.

Treatment

Hemiplegia

Specific exercise in the hydrotherapy pool has little to offer the patient with hemiplegia. All efforts to rehabilitate him are best channelled into physiotherapy on dry land, occupational therapy and speech therapy if required. In water, which as a movement medium provides less stability for the patient, associated reactions occur very easily, preventing purposeful movement being re-educated. Any movement by another person in the pool or that made by the patient himself causes disturbance of the water with turbulence. This is very likely to further disrupt the posture and balance of the patient, causing associated reactions to supercede, thus further preventing the patient from gaining control.

Swimming can be a useful recreational pursuit for the hemiplegic patient if he is generally fit enough, and sessions in a pool to teach the use of head control in the water, to develop confidence in the water and to learn suitable swimming strokes are valuable for the patient who is wishing to use this form of leisure.

Head injury

The degree of neurological involvement and resultant spasticity are, of course, enormously variable following trauma to the head, and every patient will present with different neurological signs. However, the comments concerning pool therapy for the hemiplegic patient relate also to head injured patients.

It is sometimes of value to treat a patient after head injury in the pool if he demonstrates particular tightness of the trunk, and also if there is weakness in any muscle groups. Care must be taken not to increase spasticity by demanding too much effort from the patient. It is not possible to discuss treatment in any detail as the whole programme will depend upon the assessment of the patient and the specific physical problems in terms of weakness, spasticity, incoordination, etc., and the most appropriate means to use, which could exclude pool therapy.

Multiple sclerosis

As, in the majority of cases, patients with multiple sclerosis have a poor tolerance of heat, treatment in the warm hydrotherapy pool is usually contra-indicated. Extreme fatigue occurs after only the briefest pool session and the psychological advantage to the patient of being able to generally move more easily in the pool is totally negated by the loss of ability which follows in the few hours after a session.

There are always exceptions to any such general comment, particularly when considering a condition such as multiple sclerosis. The authors have treated such patients in the pool with no untoward effect, but it is their opinion that these have been the patients who are not so subject to frequent exacerbations and remissions and whose condition is relatively stable.

However, pool therapy in such cases needs to be undemanding with movements performed slowly and with frequent rests. Walking and associated gait activities are perhaps the most helpful. It is, on balance, best if the patient is not referred for pool therapy, and the physiotherapist should do her best to prevent medical staff from suggesting it and certainly to refuse requests from physiotherapy colleagues unless the psychological effect is seen to be of paramount importance in the patient's management. Only then may it be worth a trial two or three sessions.

ACQUIRED IMMUNE DEFICIENCY SYNDROME (AIDS)

This syndrome is caused by a virus known as HTLV III which is epidemiologically similar to hepatitis. From information available to date, a large percentage of people who acquire the virus go on to develop AIDS. All carriers are thought to be infectious.

The spread of the HTLV III virus occurs through blood, blood products and by sexual contact. There is no evidence of airborne transmission as by coughing or sneezing. The presence of antibodies does not indicate immunity to the virus, but does indicate that the person concerned carries the virus and may infect others.

The HTLV III virus causes illness by lowering the body resistance to infection by damage to the immune system. It depletes the number of T helper lymphocytes which particularly defend the body against viral, fungal and parasitic infections and some types of tumours.

Pool therapy

Patients with AIDS may be referred for pool therapy because of generalised weakness and loss of mobility. Providing there are no skin abrasions or wounds, the patient can be treated in the hydrotherapy pool to great advantage (p. 51). A generalised programme of strengthening and mobilising exercises using patterns of movement as in the Bad Ragaz method can be given and progressed accordingly. Trunk patterns in supine will be important, but should be given slowly and possibly initially through only part of range. These patients will very often be extremely weak and care must be taken not to cause undue fatigue. Lower extremity patterns can be added and gait activities will be found useful.

As well as the physical benefit derived from pool therapy these patients will also benefit psychologically. There is still some lack of understanding by the general public about AIDS and the ways in which it can and cannot be transmitted. There is also a certain stigma attached to patients with this condition and physiotherapists should make sure that no discussion concerning their patients should take place in the hydrotherapy department where it may be overheard, in the same way that confidentiality is respected about any patient's condition.

REFERENCES

Adams J C 1983 Outline of fractures, 8th edn. Churchill Livingstone, Edinburgh
Bannister R 1985 Brain's Clinical neurology, 6th Edn. Oxford University Press, Oxford
Bulstrode S J, Barefoot J, Harrison R A, Clarke A K 1986 The role of passive stretching in the treatment of ankylosing spondylitis. British Journal of Rheumatology
Chusid J G 1985 Correlative neuroanatomy and functional neurology, 19th edn. Lange Medical Publications, Los Altos, California
Davies P 1985 Steps to follow. Springer-Verlag, Berlin and Heidelberg
Hayward R 1980 Essentials of neurosurgery. Blackwell Scientific Publications, Oxford
Moll J M H 1980 Ankylosing spondylitis. Churchill Livingstone, Edinburgh
Zuckerman A J 1986 AIDS and swimming pools. British Medical Journal 293:221

9

Spas and spa treatments

A spa is a resort where a natural spring, having unusual properties, is used therapeutically. These resorts are often situated in places of outstanding natural beauty, which also have a good climate. Before a mineral spring is considered to be medicinal from the spa point of view, it must have a higher content of minerals than normal drinking water, or its temperature must be above 20 °C.

Although the spas in Britain were highly developed from the eighteenth century until early in the present century, there remains now only a vestige of what once existed and their final decline is often attributed to the advent of the National Health Service in 1948.

This has not been the case, however, on the continent of Europe or in the USSR, where spas still play an important part in the health care of these countries. Their role is not only in the treatment of the sick, but also in the field of preventative medicine, and every year the governments of these countries spend an equivalent of millions of pounds to pay for the treatment of their nationals in the spa centres.

For the disabled, the best spas offer all the benefits of the modern rehabilitation centre besides providing the traditional water treatments of the spa.

There is, in many spas, a 'season' which is usually from May until October, and some spas are virtually closed during the rest of the year. Other spa towns have become attractive during the closed season to other visitors and have developed as conference towns.

Since besides treatment the spa offers rest and relaxation, there is often the opportunity to follow athletic, sporting or intellectual activities so that theatres, concert halls and recreation centres may form part of the spa complex.

Emphasis is often placed on diet and the regulation of daily regimen, and some spa physicians give this equal importance with physical rehabilitation. There are some spas where treatment is specific to the gastrointestinal tract and the doctors specialise in the treatment of gastric, intestinal, hepatic diseases, obesity and diabetes.

Other spas treat only respiratory conditions and are situated in forested or mountainous areas where graded outdoor exercise in the form of forest walks is as much part of the treatment as the mineral water inhalations.

Not unnaturally, when bathing forms an integral part of the 'water cure', the treatment of skin conditions is one of the areas where spas have claimed success so that there are spas which attract both dermatologists and their patients.

Drinking the water at spas has always been part of the 'cure' and many establishments have elaborate and beautiful pump rooms which, besides dispensing the mineral water, act as meeting places and are the focal point for the social life of the resort.

Treatment will be given by physiotherapists or sometimes by relatively untrained personnel who are technicians giving treatment under the direction of the physician in charge. In the better spas the true rehabilitation type of treatment will be given by qualified physiotherapists, but in others the patients are treated only by technicians. Physiotherapists who may consider working in a spa should, therefore, make very careful enquiries about the exact nature of the job before accepting a post. Whilst some spa establishments, for example those at Leukerbad and Bad Ragaz, have achieved international reputations for their progressive attitude towards rehabilitation, others would have little to offer the physiotherapist looking for professional development.

Some spas will be primarily business concerns, whilst others will be primarily medical, but all will have a physician in attendance.

Patients visiting spas will usually stay in a hotel and visit the treatment centre daily. Sometimes the hotels are connected to the spas, and in some larger spas, the hotels have their own treatment rooms in the hotel with water piped directly from the spring.

The patient will probably spend between one and four hours having treatment each day, with several hours put aside for rest, and the remainder of his time will be spent in some other diversion as mentioned above. It has to be said that a spa may often be chosen on the merits of its diversions rather than the efficacy of its waters, but if a person's main reason for visiting the spa is to have a holiday whilst at the same time promoting his health and well-being this is, perhaps, allowable.

There cannot be a method of application of water to the human body which has not been thought of and utilised at some spa. Water is applied externally by immersion, douches, sprays and massage, as steam vapour, or mixed with mud or peat and applied hot to the skin. It is applied internally by irrigation of the colon, rectum, vagina, mouth and nasal cavities as well as by inhalation. All these methods of application have a rationale for their use, some sound and others rather imaginative, and claim successful remedial use.

A few of these spa treatments are described in this chapter and are those which the physiotherapist may find herself required to do if working in such an establishment.

TREATMENTS

Vichy spray massage (Fig. 9.1)

This is a treatment not usually encountered in British hospitals, although it may be found in private medical establishments. In continental spas, however, it is still in common use.

The apparatus consists of a shallow trough mounted on legs which bring it to about waist height. Above the trough five to six pairs of 'rose' sprays, which are similar to shower heads, deliver water at 2 to 4 lb/sq in and at a temperature of about 39 °C.

The patient lies in the trough beneath the sprays, whilst the physiotherapist performs massage manipulations to all four limbs, back and abdomen, the patient turning from prone to supine lying as necessary. Where appropriate, the massage is followed by passive movements to the joints. The whole procedure lasts for about twenty minutes and is followed by a shower at neutral temperature and then a rest period, usually in a 'pack' (see p. 67).

Fig. 9.1 Vichy spray massage

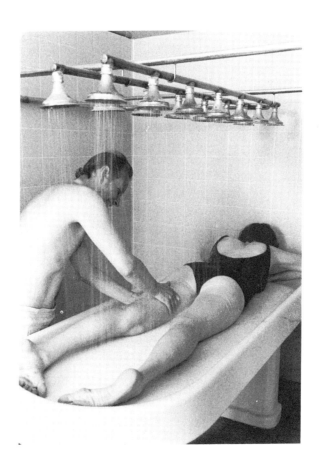

Manipulations

Kneading, finger-kneading around joints and skin rolling are among the manipulations usually used in this treatment. Percussive massage is not used, and although wringing movements may be used by a practised masseur, they are difficult since the operator's hands tend to slip on the wet skin. Effleurage is, for the same reason, modified to a lighter, quicker movement known as 'skin polishing'.

Effects

The percussive effect of the jets of water produces a marked erythema and this, together with the massage, has been claimed to increase the general circulation, break down adhesions around joints and reduce to fibrous thickenings in chronic fibrositis and panniculitis.

The underwater douche

Sometimes called the undercurrent douche, this is a local treatment used on a muscle group or on one joint, and since it calls for the part being treated to be beneath the surface of the water, it is usually used in conjunction with pool therapy. It is one of the few spa treatments which may still be found in some modern hospital hydrotherapy departments.

The apparatus consists of a flexible hose connected to the hot and cold supply via a thermostatic mixing valve, and has a thermometer and a pressure gauge incorporated. At the end of the hose, which is long enough to reach well into the pool and below the surface, is a nozzle which has a bore of about 10 mm. Through this nozzle is delivered a jet of water between 2 and 5 °C above the temperature of the pool and at a pressure of 10 lb/sq in.

The part to be treated is positioned below the surface of the pool and the jet of water moved over the area in a circular motion. The jet may be thought of as replacing the fingers or hand of the physiotherapist when performing conventional massage. Initially the tip of the nozzle is held at a distance of about 10 cm from the skin, but may need to be moved closer or further away in order to increase or decrease the pressure.

The mechanical effects are the same as those of kneading (petrissage) manipulations to the muscles, or finger-kneading around joints, and this, combined with the warmth of the water, provides an effective method of relaxation of protective muscle spasm or assisting in the mobilisation of stiff joints.

The underwater douche is nowadays usually used as a preparatory treatment to exercises in water rather than as a treatment in its own right.

The contrast douche

This general treatment consists of playing alternate hot and cold jets of water over the body in a prescribed pattern. The hot jet is used first and this is followed by the cold jet which follows the same course, but is applied for a shorter time. During the treatment, the patient stands in a needle spray, the water of which is kept at a neutral temperature of about 37 °C.

(A needle spray consists of a series of horse-shoe shaped pipes fixed horizontally one above the other at a distance apart of about 0.25 m. Each of the pipes has approximately 100 small holes through which fine jets of water, i.e. needles, play onto the patient's skin from the level of his ankles to his shoulders.)

The hot and cold jets are operated by the physiotherapist from a distance of about 3 m. The hot jet is thermostatically controlled and can be set to a temperature between 38 ° and 45 °C, whilst the cold is usually used directly from the mains at a temperature between 13 ° and 22 °C. Pressures between 10 and 20 lb/sq in are used, but it is usual to have the cold jet at a slightly higher pressure than the hot jet.

Procedure

The patient stands in the needle spray with his back to the operator. Starting at the ankle the therapist plays a hot jet slowly up the patient's right leg to the buttocks and then describes a small circle over the gluteal muscles. The jet then moves up the patient's spine across the right shoulder and down the arm to the hand. The jet then moves back onto the leg, down to the ankle. This is then repeated using the cold jet, but at a speed three or four times faster than that used for the hot jet.

The same procedure is applied to the left side and after three alternate douchings to each side the patient turns to face the operator and the front is treated in the same way.

Whilst the jets are being used, the force may be broken by the physiotherapist touching the jet with the forefinger as it leaves the nozzle. This 'broken' jet is used over the whole of the front of the patient and over the posterior aspect of his arms and calves.

This is a rather rigorous treatment still used in some spas where it is hoped to increase the general circulation, but it is contra-indicated in patients with cardiac conditions, high blood pressure and varicose veins.

Whirlpool baths

These are warm or hot baths in which the water is agitated by compressed air or by paddles positioned at the bottom of the bath beneath a protective grille. Some baths may have both methods of agitating the water and are usually designed specifically for treating upper limbs or lower limbs.

The working temperature of the water is usually between 37° and 43 °C, although temperatures up to 48 °C may be used if appropriate and if the condition of the skin and the superficial circulation allow it. The warmth, combined with the gentle massaging effect of the water, stimulates the skin and brings about an improvement in the circulation, and the constant mechanical stimulus of the bubbles on the sensory nerve endings results in a decrease in pain.

Because of these combined effects, whirlpool baths have been found to be particularly useful in the treatment of post-traumatic pain and swelling in hands and feet. The treatment consists of immersing the part in the whirlpool with the agitator switched on and allowing the patient to get used to it for about five minutes. The patient then performs appropriate mobilising exercises whilst the hand or foot is still immersed.

The whirlpool bath has been much used in physical therapy departments in the USA, but in Britain was largely confined to the spa establishments which have now almost disappeared. There does, however, seem to be a renewal of interest in this form of treatment.

The aeration bath

The aeration bath consists of an ordinary domestic type of bath into the bottom of which have been fitted a series of perforated pipes which are connected to an electric air-pump. Above the pipes is a slatted wooden platform upon which the patient reclines.

The patient is placed in the bath which has been three-quarters filled with water at a temperature between 35° and 37 °C. When the patient has been made comfortable, the pump is switched on and the air which is pushed through the pipes emerges as thousands of small air bubbles which rise to the surface of the bath. As the bubbles rise they give a continuous gentle mechanical stimulation to the skin, giving a general sedative and relaxing feeling to the patient.

Hot packs

These are commercially made 'mud' packs consisting of a thick cotton material envelope filled with an inert inorganic substance such as Fullers' earth which gives the pack a high thermal capacity. The envelope is divided into pockets or compartments by rows of stitching which keep the filling evenly spread through the length of the pack and so ensure that the heat is uniformly distributed.

These packs, even when used daily, will give many months of service and are clean and easy to use. They are heated in a thermostatically controlled cabinet called a hydrocollator, and the recommended temperature for use is 70 °C.

The pack is applied to the patient after folding it in a large Terry towel in such a way that between six and eight layers of towel are interposed between the pack and the patient's skin. It is then covered over with a sheet of polythene, which helps to retain the heat and also prevents the couch becoming damp.

Since the heat from these packs comes through the towels rather slowly, it may take several minutes to reach a peak, and on no account should the patient be left during this period until the physiotherapist is certain that the pack will not get any hotter.

The usual tests, instructions and warnings are given as they would be for any heat treatment.

These packs may be purchased in several shapes and sizes which are made to suit application to various parts of the body, or they can be made up by the hospital linen room to the physiotherapist's requirements.

Hot packs are just another form of localised heat available to the physiotherapist, and are used to decrease pain prior to exercise rather than being regarded as a treatment in their own right. Many patients, however, feel that moist heat is more soothing to painful joints than infra-red and certainly this method has the advantage, when treating joints, of heating circumferentially rather than only on one surface.

Peat or mud baths

In England, peat which is suitable for therapeutic purposes is found in Harrogate and Buxton. The dry peat is mixed with water and steam heated, and is then transferred to a special bath. The temperature of the peat is between 39 °C and 40 °C, and the patient remains in the bath for 10 to 20 minutes. Following the bath the patient showers with the water temperature between 37 °C and 38 °C, and is then packed and rests for forty minutes.

Effects

The major effects are those of a rise in body temperature and the relief of pain, particularly in chronic joint conditions.

The design and use of tanks

Whilst it is widely accepted that pool therapy is an invaluable element in the treatment programme of many patients, there are still many hospitals and centres which do not have hydrotherapy pools. This may be due to a number of reasons, but most usually those of lack of space and of finance. It may also happen that in a particular hospital such treatment may be appropriate for only a small group of patients. Therefore, the cost of building and maintaining a treatment pool as described in Chapters 3 and 4 is unacceptable.

In these circumstances a specially designed tank such as a Hubbard tank can be installed which will enable patients to be treated in water, albeit with certain limitations.

The Hubbard tank is keyhole or butterfly shaped and is most usually made of stainless steel. The top of the tank is approximately one meter from the floor, and the shape and appearance is shown in Figure 9.2.

The tank is filled and emptied as required and, therefore, a plant for circulation, filtration, heating and chlorinating of the water is not necessary. However, it may be felt that the water should be disinfected, and chlorination by hand is effective as is also the use of other agents such as Chlorhexidine.

If required, a whirlpool motor can be fitted to the tank and the water agitated to achieve the effects previously described under 'whirlpools'.

The patient enters the tank either by steps over the edge or by a stretcher and hoist, usually the latter.

Because of the shape of the tank, when the patient lies in supine there is clearance for hip and shoulder abduction and when the patient is in side- lying, full range flexion and extension of hip and knee is possible, as is full elevation and extension of the shoulder.

It is only possible for one patient to be treated in the tank at a time and the physiotherapist remains on the outside. However, she has ease of control of the patient and can provide fixation for the patient, and resist or assist movement as required.

Fig. 9.2 The 'Arjo' tank with hydraulic hoist. (Reproduced with permission from Arjo Hospital Equipment Ltd, 1986)

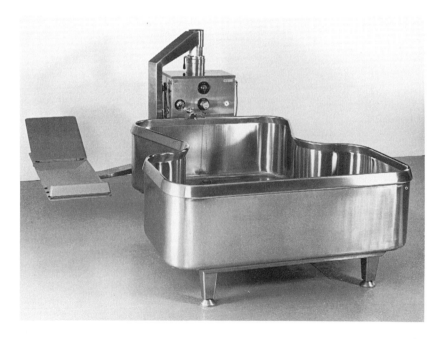

It is particularly useful to have a shaped tank such as a Hubbard tank in a Burns Unit. The tank can be filled with normal saline or the water disinfected with an alternative agent. With immersion of the patient in the tank, dressings are much more easily removed, and early movements to joints underlying burnt or grafted tissue can be encouraged.

REFERENCES

Baruch S 1950 An epitome of hydrotherapy. W B Saunders, London
Calthrop L C E 1931 Hydrotherapy and physiotherapy. W Heinemann, London
Le Quesne R M, Granville M, 1946 Hydrotherapy. Cassel, London
Licht S (ed) 1963 Medical hydrology. E. Licht, New Haven, Connecticut

Index

Accidents, 45
Acidity, see pH
Acquired Immune Deficiency
    Syndrome, see AIDS
Adjustment of resistance, varying
    shape, 54–55
Aeration bath, 176
Aides, see Helpers
AIDS, 51, 169–170
Airline jacket, see Flotation jacket
Alarm system, 21, 49
    testing, 49
Algicide, 8
Alkalinity, see pH
Ambu bag, 48
Ankylosing spondylitis, 137, 142–147
    group treatment, 146
    neck movements in, 147
    underwater swimming in, 146
    vital capacity in, 142–143
Anterior poliomyelitis, 160–161
    Bad Ragaz in, 162
Archimedes principle, application,
    58–59
    definition, 58
Architects, 1
Athletes foot, see Tinea pedis

Back-washing, 4, 5–6
Bacteriological sampling, 41–43
Bad Ragaz method, 75, 155, 157, 159,
    162
    advantages-disadvantages, 76–77
    distal holds in, 92
    in rheumatoid arthritis, 150
    lower limb, 94–102
    manual contact, 76
    patterns and technique, 91–119
    proximal holds in, 91–92
    rationale, 91–92
    resistances produced, 93
    size of pool required, 77
    stabilisations, 102–103, 112
    trunk patterns, 104–113
    upper limb patterns, 114–118

Balls, 31
Baquacil, 8
Bathing costumes, provision of, 32
Bathing load, 49
Bats, see Paddles
Bays, 13
Bleach, household, 6
    laundry, 6
Blood pressure, 51, 73
Body supports, 29
    see also Flotation jackets
Bow wave, 53
Breakpoint, 37
Bridos, 6
Bromine, 7
Bronchial wheezing, 9
Brook's airway, 48
Bulbar paralysis, 161
Buoyancy, 58–59
Buoyancy aids, 29–30
Buoyancy, centre of, 59

Calcium hypochlorite, 5–6, 7
Calorifier, 2, 4,
Cardiac arrest, 48
Catheters 72
Caustic soda, 40
Centre of buoyancy, 59
Chemicals, storage of, 47
Chloramines, 37
Chlorinating agent, 2, 38
Chlorinating pump, 2
Chlorination, hand, 7, 43
Chlorinator, 6
Chlorine, 6
Chlorine donor, 6
Chlorine levels, 36–37, 49
    monitoring, 36–40
    procedure for testing, 38
Chlorine resistant organisms, 43
Chlorine, combined, 37
    acceptable level of, 37
    free residual, 36
    gaseous, 6
    total, 38

Chloro-iso-cyanurate, 6, 7
Chloros, 6, 22
Cholera, 72
Circulating pump, 3
Clothing and linen, storage, 33–34
Coliform organisms, 41
Collars, see Neck supports
Combined chlorine, see Chlorine,
    combined
Comparator, 38
Condom drainage, 72
Contra-indications to pool therapy,
    65–71
Contract-relax, 77
Contrast douche, 175
Crohn's disease, 147
Cubicles, changing, 20

Density, 58
Di-ethyl p-phenylene diamine (DPD),
    38
Di-halo, 7
Diatoms, 5
Dosing pump, 3, 7
    cleaning, 4
Drag, 91
Dressing gowns, 32
Drowning, 48
Dry acid, 40
Dry dock 13
Dysentry, 72

Epilepsy, 73
Evaporation 63

Fail-safe device, 22
Fear of water, 73
Filter, 4–6
    bed, 5
    diatomaceous earth, 5
    disposable cartridge, 5
    sand/gravel, 5
First aid, 49
Flaccid paralysis, 160
    use of splints, 31

Floats, neck, *see* Neck supports
plastazote, 29
polystyrene, 28
sizes of, 28
Floor drains, 24
Floor, changing cubicles, 24
pool, 23
pool room, 46
pool, adjustable, 26
glazed tiled, 23
non-slip tiled, 23
showers, 24
Flooring, 23–24
Flotation aids, *see* Buoyancy aids
Flotation jacket, 29–30
upthrust of, 30
Folliculitis, *see* Swimming pool rash
Footbath, 22
Footwear, 47
pool area, 32
Fractures, 153–156
lower limb, 153–156
upper limb, 156–157
vertebrae, 158

Gait cycle, 124–126
pelvic rotation, 126
pelvic tilt, 126–127
re-education of elements, 133
stance phase, 124–125
swing phase, 126
Gait exercises, 133
Gait in water, 127–128
stance phase, 127
swing phase, 127–128
Gait re-education, 121–135
anterior poliomyelitis, 163
effect of speed, 133
fractures, 155
manual resistance, 132
osteoarthrosis, 141
plaiting, 134
standing activities, 128–130
standing balance, 130–131
stride length, 134
use of hand rails, 131
use of turbulence, 130
walking activities, 131–132
weight transference, 134
Gantry, *see* Hoist
Group treatment, 76–77
in ankylosing spondylitis, 146
Guillain-Barré syndrome, 160

Haemodilution, 71
Half-plinth, *see* pool plinth
Halogens, 7
Hand chlorination, procedure, 47
Hand rails, 22–23, 46
position in pool, 27
size of, 23
strength of, 23
use in gait re-education, 131
Head injuries, 167
Health and safety, 41–51

Heat reclamation system, 9
Heater, *see* Calorifier
Heel cup, 123
Helpers, in the pool, 35
Hemiplegia, 167
Hexachlorathene, 22
Hip exercises, 78–80
Hip stretching, in osteoarthrosis, 140
Hoist, 14–20
chairs, 14–20
compressed air, 14, 20
electrical, 14
hydraulic, 14–18
bleeding, 16
faulty seals, 16
faulty washers, 16
operation of, 16
principle of, 14
maintenance, 45
mechanical, 14, 19
overhead, 16
slings, 18
stretcher, 14–20
Hold-relax, 143
Hot cupboard, 34
Hot packs, 176
Hubbard tank, 51, 72, 177–179
Hydrogen peroxide, 8
Hydrostatic pressure, 60
Hygrometer, 62
Hyperchlorination, 40, 42, 43
Hypertension, 70
Hypertonic conditions, 166–169
Hypotonus, 160

Immersion, 65
effect on blood pressure, 70
effect on body fluids, 60, 71
effect on cardiac output, 70
effect on diastolic filling, 70–71
effect on haemoglobin, 71
effect on kidneys, 71
effect on oedema, 60–61
effect on packed cell volume, 71
effect on respiration, 61
effect on stroke volume, 70
Incontinence, of faeces, 72
of urine, 72
Infected wounds
Inflatable rings, *see* Buoyancy aids
Intra-articular injections, pool after, 151
Iso-cyanurate, granules, 7
tablets, 7

Knee exercises, 82

Laminectomy, 158–159
Latent heat, 62
Leg length, discrepancy in, 123
Leonard valve, *see* Thermostatic mixing valve
Leukerbad, 146
Linen, 31–34
Lovibond, *see* Comparator

Manual resistance, use in gait re-education, 132
Masons wet/dry hygrometer, 62
Microbiology, 41–43
Microbiology samples, frequency, 42
procedure for taking, 42
refrigeration of, 42
Movement through water, 53–55
Mud baths, 177
Multiple sclerosis, 167
Muscular dystrophy, 160, 163

National Ankylosing Spondylitis Society, 146
Needle bath, 48
Neurological conditions, 160–170
Nitrogen trichloride, 37
Normal gait, 124

Opsite, 51
Osteoarthritis, *see* Osteoarthrosis
Osteoarthrosis, 138–142
Bad Ragaz in, 139
hip stretching, 140
increasing range of movement, 139
relief of pain, 138
relief of spasm, 139
strengthening muscle, 141
Otitis externa, 41
Overshoes, *see* Footwear
Oxygen cylinder, 48
Ozone, 8–9

pH level, 49
adjustment of, 40
monitoring of, 38–40
optimum, 37
procedure for testing, 38
Packing, procedure, 67
Paddles, 31
use of, 55
Parallel bars, 26, 46
Partial weight-bearing, 121–123, 154
quantification, 122
standing, 122
Passive stretching, 140–141
Patients, handling, 152
Peat baths, 177
Periodic Table, 7
Phenol red, 38
Physical principles, 53
Physiological effects of pool therapy, 65–71
Plantar warts, *see* Verrucae
Plinths, 46
Plombiere sheets, *see* Pool gowns
Polyneuropathy, 160
Pool gowns, dimensions for making, 33
Pool lifts, *see* Hoists
Pool records, importance of, 42
Pool room, cleaning, 50
temperature of, 51
Pool size, for Bad Ragaz, 77
Pool steps, 22